# Table of Contents

## Vegan Keto Cookbook
*Over 190 High-Fat Low-Carb Plant-Based Recipes to Shed Fat and Heal You from the Inside Out*

**INTRODUCTION AND OVERVIEW AS A KETO VEGAN** ............................................................. 3
    MAKE USE OF LOW-CARB SUBSTITUTIONS ............................................................. 9
    SELECT KETO-FRIENDLY SWEETENERS ............................................................. 10
    KETOGENIC VEGETABLE CHOICES ............................................................. 11
    GET YOUR NUTRIENTS FROM VEGGIES ............................................................. 13

**CHAPTER 1: MORNING AND BRUNCH SPECIALTIES** ............................................................. 17
    BEGIN A KETOGENIC ROUTINE ............................................................. 17
        *Bulletproof Coffee* ............................................................. 17
        *Bulletproof Tea* ............................................................. 18
    PANCAKE TIME ............................................................. 18
        *Cinnamon Roll Pancakes* ............................................................. 18
        *Coconut Pancakes* ............................................................. 20
        *Crispy Flaxseed Waffles* ............................................................. 21
        *Flaxseed Pancakes* ............................................................. 23
        *Scallion Pancakes* ............................................................. 24
    OTHER DELICIOUS CHOICES ............................................................. 25
        *Almonds and Chips Breakfast Cereal* ............................................................. 25
        *Avocado – Carrot and Tahini Breakfast Bowl* ............................................................. 26
        *Bagel Thins for Breakfast* ............................................................. 27
        *Berry and Nut Cereal* ............................................................. 28
        *Blueberry Breakfast Cake – Flourless and Gluten-Free* ............................................................. 29
        *Bran Muffins – Gluten-Free* ............................................................. 30
        *Breakfast Quiche* ............................................................. 31
        *Cinnamon Roll Muffins* ............................................................. 32
        *Macadamia Breakfast Bars* ............................................................. 34
        *Maple Walnut Breakfast Cereal* ............................................................. 34
        *Minty Eggplant Hash Browns* ............................................................. 35
        *Muesli in the Raw* ............................................................. 36
        *Peanut Butter Breakfast Cereal* ............................................................. 37
        *Psyllium Breakfast Mix* ............................................................. 37
        *Pumpkin Pie Breakfast Cereal* ............................................................. 38
        *Scrambled Tofu* ............................................................. 39
        *Seed and Nut-Packed Bread* ............................................................. 39
        *Vanilla and Turmeric Breakfast Cereal* ............................................................. 41
    OATMEAL AND PORRIDGE FAVORITES ............................................................. 42
        *Berries and Hemp Seeds* ............................................................. 42
        *Blueberry Porridge* ............................................................. 42
        *Fudge Oatmeal* ............................................................. 44
    OVERNIGHT OAT OPTIONS ............................................................. 45
        *Alternative #1: Vanilla Oats: The Base* ............................................................. 45

  *Alternative #2: Pumpkin Spice Latte Overnight Oats* ...... 46
  *Alternative #3: Fudge Overnight Oats* ...... 46
 PORRIDGE OPTIONS ...... 47
  *Delicious Plain Porridge* ...... 47
  *Porridge with Cinnamon and Hemp Hearts* ...... 48

# CHAPTER 2: DELICIOUS MEALS AND SALADS ...... 50

 MEALS ...... 50
  *Asparagus and Mushrooms with Cauliflower Risotto* ...... 50
  *Asparagus and Tofu Stir Fry* ...... 51
  *Broccoli Noodles and Tofu* ...... 52
  *Cauliflower Tabbouleh* ...... 54
  *Collard Green Wraps* ...... 55
  *Crispy Tofu and Cauliflower Rice* ...... 55
  *Eggplant Lasagna* ...... 57
  *Falafel with Tahini Sauce* ...... 58
  *French Style Ratatouille* ...... 60
  *Green Panini* ...... 62
  *Sesame Tofu and Eggplant* ...... 63
 SALADS ...... 64
  *Arugula and Blueberry Salad* ...... 64
  *Asian Zucchini Salad* ...... 65
  *Asparagus and Artichoke Salad* ...... 66
  *Avocado and Greens Salad* ...... 67
  *Avocado Papaya Salad* ...... 68
  *Bell Pepper and Asparagus Salad* ...... 68
  *Caesar Vegan Salad* ...... 69
  *Courgette Salad and Herbed Vinaigrette* ...... 70
  *Eggplant Salad* ...... 71
  *Kale Salad and Blueberry Dressing* ...... 72
  *Lemony Brussel Sprout Salad* ...... 74
  *Pear and Dates with Special Cider Dressing* ...... 74
  *Pecan Cauliflower Salad* ...... 76
  *Simple Green Salad with Lemon Vinaigrette* ...... 76
  *Sun-Dried Tomato Salad and Cider Dressing* ...... 77
  *Thai Peanut Zucchini Noodle Salad* ...... 78

# CHAPTER 3: HEALTHY SOUPS – STEWS AND CHOWDER ...... 81

 *Beetroot Ginger Soup* ...... 81
 *Broccoli and Cauliflower Soup* ...... 82
 *Cabbage and Beet Soup* ...... 83
 *Chili – Vegan Style* ...... 84
 *Chilled Minty Avocado Soup* ...... 85
 *Creamy Avocado Soup* ...... 86
 *Creamy Red Gazpacho Soup* ...... 87
 *Creamy Tomato Soup* ...... 88
 *Ginger Cauliflower Stew* ...... 90
 *Mushroom Soup* ...... 91
 *Red Onion Soup* ...... 93

  *Spanish Soup* .................................................................................................................. *94*
  *Spinach and Turnip Soup* ............................................................................................ *94*
  *Superfood Keto Soup* ................................................................................................... *95*
  *Thai Pumpkin Soup* ...................................................................................................... *97*
  *Turmeric Cabbage Soup* .............................................................................................. *98*
  *Zucchini Basil Soup* ..................................................................................................... *99*

**CHAPTER 4: VEGAN CREAMS - SAUCES AND DIPS** .................................................................... **101**
  *Avocado Mayo* ............................................................................................................ *101*
  *Barbecue Sauce* .......................................................................................................... *101*
  *Coconut Whipped Cream* .......................................................................................... *102*
  *Eggplant Bruschetta* .................................................................................................. *103*
  *Guacamole* ................................................................................................................. *104*
  *Hummus and Avocado* .............................................................................................. *104*
  *Ketchup* ...................................................................................................................... *105*
  *Lemon and Jalapeno Cream Sauce* ........................................................................... *106*
  *Mayo – Vegan Style* ................................................................................................... *107*
  *Nutella Spread* ........................................................................................................... *108*
  *Peanut Sauce* ............................................................................................................. *109*
  *Portobello Mushroom Bruschetta* ............................................................................ *110*
  *Slow-Cooked Summer Bruschetta* ............................................................................ *110*
  *Spinach Avocado Dip* ................................................................................................ *111*
  *Tahini and Cilantro Sauce* ......................................................................................... *113*
  *Tofu or Seitan Marinades* ......................................................................................... *114*
  *Vegan Sour Cream* .................................................................................................... *117*
  *Veggie Salsa* ............................................................................................................... *118*

**CHAPTER 5: APPETIZERS – SIDES AND SNACKS** ........................................................................ **119**
 SIDES ..................................................................................................................................... 119
  *Basil Zoodles and Olives* ........................................................................................... *119*
  *Beetroot and Pesto Noodles* ..................................................................................... *120*
  *Brussels Sprouts and Cashew Dip* ............................................................................. *120*
  *Cabbage Slaw* ............................................................................................................ *121*
  *Carrot and Zucchini Noodles in Thai Sauce* ............................................................. *122*
  *Cauliflower and Artichoke Couscous* ....................................................................... *123*
  *Cauliflower Bites with Ranch Dip* ............................................................................. *124*
  *Cherry Tomatoes and Zucchini Pasta* ....................................................................... *125*
  *Chili and Coconut Cauliflower Rice* .......................................................................... *126*
  *Coconut Cauliflower Rice* ......................................................................................... *127*
  *Creamy Curry Low-Carb Noodle Bowl* ..................................................................... *127*
  *Edamame Kelp Noodles* ............................................................................................ *129*
  *Garlicky Mushrooms* ................................................................................................. *130*
  *Grilled Eggplant and Zucchini* ................................................................................... *131*
  *Indian Curried Cauliflower* ....................................................................................... *132*
  *Kelp Noodles with Peanut Butter Sauce* .................................................................. *133*
  *Lime and Chili Carrot Noodles* .................................................................................. *133*
  *Mediterranean Spaghetti Squash* ............................................................................ *134*
  *Mushroom, Broccoli, and Squash Noodles* .............................................................. *135*
  *Nutty Pesto Zucchini* ................................................................................................. *136*

- Pesto Kelp Noodles ............................................................................................................... 137
- Roasted Beetroot Noodles .................................................................................................... 138
- Roasted Broccoli .................................................................................................................. 139
- Roasted Green Cabbage ....................................................................................................... 140
- Roasted Kale and Squash ..................................................................................................... 141
- Spaghetti Squash .................................................................................................................. 142
- Sriracha Grilled Asparagus .................................................................................................. 143
- Teriyaki Grilled Eggplant .................................................................................................... 144
- Tofu Pizza Sticks .................................................................................................................. 144
- Turnip Fries .......................................................................................................................... 145
- Turnip and Courgette Hash Browns ..................................................................................... 146
- Zucchini Noodles and Avocado Sauce ................................................................................. 147

## SNACK TIME TREATS .................................................................................................................. 148
- Carrot Cake Bites ................................................................................................................. 148
- Chocolate Granola ................................................................................................................ 149
- Chocolate Protein Bars ......................................................................................................... 150
- Cinnamon Granola ............................................................................................................... 151
- Coconut and Peanut Butter Balls ......................................................................................... 151
- Fudge Balls .......................................................................................................................... 152
- Loaded Nut-Packed Coconut Granola ................................................................................. 153
- Mushroom Chips .................................................................................................................. 154
- Pecan and Maple Fat Bars .................................................................................................... 156
- Peanut Butter Fat Bombs ..................................................................................................... 156
- Peanut Tofu Wrap ................................................................................................................ 157
- Roasted Radish Chips .......................................................................................................... 158
- Sweet Potato Toast ............................................................................................................... 159
- Zucchini Chips ..................................................................................................................... 160

# CHAPTER 6: DESSERTS – SMOOTHIES AND BEVERAGES ................................................ 161

## PUDDING SPECIALTIES .............................................................................................................. 161
- Avocado and Chocolate Pudding ......................................................................................... 161
- Chia Chocolate Pudding ...................................................................................................... 162
- Chia Raspberry Pudding ...................................................................................................... 163
- Chia Strawberry Pudding ..................................................................................................... 164
- Coconut Chia and Turmeric Pudding ................................................................................... 164
- Pumpkin and Peanut Butter Pudding ................................................................................... 165

## OTHER DELICIOUS DESSERTS ................................................................................................... 166
- Avocado Chocolate Mousse ................................................................................................. 166
- Banana Bread ....................................................................................................................... 167
- Cashew and Blueberry Cheesecake ..................................................................................... 168
- Chilled Avocado and Strawberry Bowl ............................................................................... 169
- Cinnamon and Pumpkin Fudge ............................................................................................ 169
- Coconut Bombs .................................................................................................................... 170
- Coconut Cupcakes ................................................................................................................ 171
- Coconut Maple Fudge .......................................................................................................... 172
- Coconut and Peanut Butter Balls ......................................................................................... 173
- Coconut and Strawberry Bars .............................................................................................. 174
- Dairy-Free Chocolate Silk Pie ............................................................................................. 174
- Lime Avocado Popsicles ...................................................................................................... 176

- *Mexican Chocolate Avocado Ice Cream* .................................................................................................. 176
- *Minty Berries in A Dish* ............................................................................................................................ 177
- *Pecan and Blueberry Crumble* ................................................................................................................. 178
- *Pumpkin Truffles* ..................................................................................................................................... 179
- *Raspberry Coconut Bark* .......................................................................................................................... 180
- *Raspberry Truffles* ................................................................................................................................... 181
- *Strawberry Ice Cream* .............................................................................................................................. 182

SMOOTHIES FOR ALMOST ANY OCCASION ........................................................................................................ 182
- *Avocado Raspberry Smoothie* ................................................................................................................. 182
- *Banana Bread and Blueberry Smoothie* .................................................................................................. 183
- *Berry Smoothie Bowl* ............................................................................................................................... 184
- *Black Currant and Strawberry Smoothie* ................................................................................................. 184
- *Blueberry Sensation* ................................................................................................................................ 185
- *Chocolate and Mint Smoothie* ................................................................................................................. 186
- *Chocolate Smoothie* ................................................................................................................................ 187
- *Cinnamon Chocolate Smoothie* ............................................................................................................... 188
- *Cinnamon Roll Smoothie* ........................................................................................................................ 188
- *Easter Time Smoothie* ............................................................................................................................. 189
- *Green Choco Smoothies* .......................................................................................................................... 190
- *Maca Almond Smoothie* .......................................................................................................................... 191
- *Minty Avocado and Spinach Smoothie* ................................................................................................... 191
- *Pumpkin and Avocado Smoothie* ............................................................................................................ 192
- *Spinach and Cucumber Smoothie* ........................................................................................................... 193

COLD BEVERAGES ............................................................................................................................................. 194
- *Green Coffee Shake* ................................................................................................................................ 194
- *Iced Blended Coffee* ................................................................................................................................ 194
- *McKeto Strawberry Milkshake* ................................................................................................................ 195

HOT BEVERAGES .............................................................................................................................................. 196
- *Coconut – Coffee Mug* ............................................................................................................................ 196
- *Creamy Hot Cocoa in the Crockpot* ........................................................................................................ 197
- *Energizing Latte* ...................................................................................................................................... 197

**A FINAL WORD** ............................................................................................................................................ 199

KEEP YOUR FINAL GOALS IN MIND WHILE ON THE KETO JOURNEY ................................................................. 203
- *More about those plateaus* ..................................................................................................................... 204
- *Benefits of Ketogenic Diet as a Vegan* .................................................................................................... 206

**CONCLUSION** .............................................................................................................................................. 208

**INDEX FOR THE RECIPES** ............................................................................................................................ 210

# Keto Diet for Beginners

*Achieve Rapid Weight Loss and Burn Fat Forever in Just 21 Days with the Ketogenic Diet - Lose Up to 21 Pounds in 3 Weeks*

**INTRODUCTION** ............................................................................................................................................ 221

**CHAPTER 1: LOW-CARB AND HIGH-FAT** ..................................................................................................... 223

BEGINNING A KETO DIET ................................................................................................................................. 224
HOW LOW IS LOW-CARB? ................................................................................................................................ 225

- Basics ..................................................................................................................................................... 225
- Macros .................................................................................................................................................. 226
- Why Try Keto? .................................................................................................................................... 228
  - *Cancer Fighter* ............................................................................................................................ 229
  - *Prevents Heart Disease* ............................................................................................................. 229
  - *Decreases Inflammation* ............................................................................................................ 230
  - *Improves Energy and Sleep* ...................................................................................................... 230
  - *Stable Uric Acid Levels* .............................................................................................................. 230
  - *Assists Gastrointestinal and Gallbladder Health* ..................................................................... 230
  - *Assists with Women's Health* ................................................................................................... 231
  - *Helps the Eyes* ............................................................................................................................ 231
  - *Help Muscle Gain and Improves Endurance* ........................................................................... 231
  - *Improves Obesity, Diabetes, and Metabolic Syndrome* ......................................................... 231

**CHAPTER 2: KETO IN STEPS** ............................................................................................................... 233
- Clean Out the Pantry ......................................................................................................................... 233
- Let's Go Shopping .............................................................................................................................. 234
- Setting up The Kitchen ...................................................................................................................... 235
- Exercise ............................................................................................................................................... 237
  - *Keto Along with Cardio* ............................................................................................................. 238
  - *Keto and Weight Lifting* ............................................................................................................ 239
  - *Exercise and Keto in Harmony* .................................................................................................. 240

**CHAPTER 3: WHAT TO EXPECT** .......................................................................................................... 241
- Side Effects of Keto ........................................................................................................................... 241
- Dangers of Keto .................................................................................................................................. 242

**CHAPTER 4: KETOSIS AND REACHING IT** .......................................................................................... 245
- Getting into Ketosis ........................................................................................................................... 245
- Fuel for the Brain ............................................................................................................................... 245
- Ketosis versus Ketoacidosis ............................................................................................................. 246
- Getting to Optimal Ketosis ............................................................................................................... 246
- How to Measure Ketosis ................................................................................................................... 247

**CHAPTER 5: WHAT TYPE IS RIGHT FOR YOU** ................................................................................... 250
- Four Kinds of Keto ............................................................................................................................. 250
  - *Standard Ketogenic Diet* ........................................................................................................... 250
  - *Targeted Ketogenic Diet* ........................................................................................................... 251
  - *Cyclical Ketogenic Diet* ............................................................................................................. 252
  - *High Protein Ketogenic Diet* ..................................................................................................... 252
  - *Muscle Maintenance* ................................................................................................................. 253
  - *How to Choose the Right Diet* .................................................................................................. 253

**CHAPTER 6: MAKING KETO WORK FOR YOU** ................................................................................... 255
- Budget ................................................................................................................................................. 255
- Traveling ............................................................................................................................................. 256
- Keto While Dining Out ...................................................................................................................... 257
- You're Not a Cook .............................................................................................................................. 258
- Holidays .............................................................................................................................................. 259

## CHAPTER 7: WHAT YOU SHOULD AND SHOULDN'T EAT .................................................................. 260
### WHAT YOU SHOULDN'T EAT .................................................................. 260
### FOODS YOU SHOULD EAT .................................................................. 261

## CHAPTER 8: IS IT RIGHT FOR YOU .................................................................. 263
### PREGNANT OR NURSING .................................................................. 263
### MEDICATION-CAUSED HYPOGLYCEMIA .................................................................. 263
### DIABETES OR BLOOD SUGAR PROBLEMS .................................................................. 264
### ON OTHER MEDICATIONS .................................................................. 264
### UNDERWEIGHT OR NUTRIENT DEFICIENT .................................................................. 264
### CHILDREN .................................................................. 265
### KIDNEY DISEASE OR STONES .................................................................. 265
### GALLSTONES OR GALL BLADDER REMOVAL .................................................................. 265
### ENZYME DEFICIENCY OR DEFECT .................................................................. 265

## CHAPTER 9: LOSE 21 POUNDS IN 21 DAYS .................................................................. 267
### WEEK ONE .................................................................. 268
#### Breakfast: .................................................................. 268
#### Lunch: .................................................................. 268
#### Dinner: .................................................................. 268
#### Snacks: .................................................................. 268
### WEEK TWO .................................................................. 279
#### Breakfast: .................................................................. 279
#### Lunch: .................................................................. 279
#### Dinner: .................................................................. 279
#### Snacks: .................................................................. 279
### WEEK THREE .................................................................. 292
#### Breakfast: .................................................................. 292
#### Lunch: .................................................................. 292
#### Dinner: .................................................................. 292
#### Snacks: .................................................................. 293

## CHAPTER 10: BREAKFAST .................................................................. 315
### PEANUT BUTTER CUP SMOOTHIE .................................................................. 315
#### What you need: .................................................................. 315
#### What you do: .................................................................. 315
### BREAKFAST BAKE .................................................................. 315
#### What you need: .................................................................. 315
#### What you do: .................................................................. 316
### MUSHROOM FRITTATA .................................................................. 317
#### What you need: .................................................................. 317
#### What you do: .................................................................. 317
### AVOCADO AND EGGS .................................................................. 318
#### What you need: .................................................................. 318
#### What you do: .................................................................. 318
### CREAMY CINNAMON SMOOTHIE .................................................................. 319
#### What you need: .................................................................. 319
#### What you do: .................................................................. 319
### EVERYTHING BAGEL .................................................................. 319

- *What you need:* ..............................................................................................319
- *What you do:* ................................................................................................320
- Nut Medley Granola ............................................................................................320
  - *What you need:* ..............................................................................................320
  - *What you do:* ................................................................................................321
- Berry Green Smoothie ........................................................................................322
  - *What you need:* ..............................................................................................322
  - *What you do:* ................................................................................................322
- Bacon Artichoke Omelet ....................................................................................323
  - *What you need:* ..............................................................................................323
  - *What you do:* ................................................................................................323

## CHAPTER 11: MAIN DISHES .................................................................................325

- Stuffed Chicken Breasts ....................................................................................325
  - *What you need:* ..............................................................................................325
  - *What you do:* ................................................................................................325
- Roasted Pork Loin with Mustard Sauce ............................................................326
  - *What you need:* ..............................................................................................326
  - *What you do:* ................................................................................................326
- Garlic-Braised Short Rib ....................................................................................327
  - *What you need:* ..............................................................................................327
  - *What you do:* ................................................................................................327
- Italian Beef Burgers ............................................................................................328
  - *What you need:* ..............................................................................................328
  - *What you do:* ................................................................................................328
- Sirloin with Compound Butter ............................................................................329
  - *What you need:* ..............................................................................................329
  - *What you do:* ................................................................................................329
- Lamb with Tomato Pesto ....................................................................................330
  - *What you need:* ..............................................................................................330
  - *What you do:* ................................................................................................331
- Lamb Chops with Kalamata Tapenade ..............................................................331
  - *What you need:* ..............................................................................................331
  - *What you do:* ................................................................................................332
- Herb Butter Scallops ..........................................................................................333
  - *What you need:* ..............................................................................................333
  - *What you do:* ................................................................................................333
- Halibut with Citrus Butter Sauce ......................................................................334
  - *What you need:* ..............................................................................................334
  - *What you do:* ................................................................................................334
- Coconut Haddock ................................................................................................335
  - *What you need:* ..............................................................................................335
  - *What you do:* ................................................................................................335

## CHAPTER 12: SIDE DISHES ...................................................................................337

- Asparagus and Walnuts ....................................................................................337
  - *What you need:* ..............................................................................................337
  - *What you do:* ................................................................................................337
- Creamed Spinach ................................................................................................338

  *What you need:* ........... 338
  *What you do:* ........... 338
 Golden Rosti ........... 339
  *What you need:* ........... 339
  *What you do:* ........... 339
 Mushrooms with Camembert ........... 340
  *What you need:* ........... 340
  *What you do:* ........... 340
 Crispy Zucchini ........... 340
  *What you need:* ........... 340
  *What you do:* ........... 341
 Cheesy Cauliflower ........... 341
  *What you need:* ........... 341
  *What you do:* ........... 341
 Cheesy Bacon Deviled Eggs ........... 342
  *What you need:* ........... 342
  *What you do:* ........... 342

## CHAPTER 13: DESSERTS, FAT BOMBS, AND EXTRAS ........... 344

 Doughnut Holes ........... 344
  *What you need:* ........... 344
  *What you do:* ........... 344
 Chocolate-Coconut Treats ........... 345
  *What you need:* ........... 345
  *What you do:* ........... 345
 Herbed Avocado Butter ........... 345
  *What you need:* ........... 346
  *What you do:* ........... 346
 Mayonnaise ........... 346
  *What you need:* ........... 346
  *What you do:* ........... 347
 Peanut Butter Cups ........... 347
  *What you need:* ........... 347
  *What you do:* ........... 348
 Peanut Butter Mousse ........... 348
  *What you need:* ........... 348
  *What you do:* ........... 348
 Strawberry Butter ........... 349
  *What you need:* ........... 349
  *What you do:* ........... 349
 Balsamic Dressing ........... 350
  *What you need:* ........... 350
  *What you do:* ........... 350
 Hollandaise ........... 351
  *What you need:* ........... 351
  *What you do:* ........... 351

## CONCLUSION ........... 353

## DESCRIPTION ........... 354

# Vegan Keto Cookbook

*Over 190 High-Fat Low-Carb Plant-Based Recipes to Shed Fat and Heal You from the Inside Out*

Tyler MacDonald

© Copyright 2019 by Tyler MacDonald - All rights reserved.

The following Book is reproduced below with the goal of providing information that is as accurate and reliable as possible. Regardless, purchasing this Book can be seen as consent to the fact that both the publisher and the author of this book are in no way experts on the topics discussed within and that any recommendations or suggestions that are made herein are for entertainment purposes only. Professionals should be consulted as needed prior to undertaking any of the action endorsed herein.

This declaration is deemed fair and valid by both the American Bar Association and the Committee of Publishers Association and is legally binding throughout the United States.

Furthermore, the transmission, duplication, or reproduction of any of the following work including specific information will be considered an illegal act irrespective of if it is done electronically or in print. This extends to creating a secondary or tertiary copy of the work or a recorded copy and is only allowed with the expressed written consent from the Publisher. All additional rights reserved.

The information in the following pages is broadly considered a truthful and accurate account of facts and as such, any inattention, use, or misuse of the information in question by the reader will render any resulting actions solely under their purview. There are no scenarios in which the publisher or the original author of this work can be in any fashion deemed liable for any hardship or damages that may befall them after undertaking information described herein.

Additionally, the information in the following pages is intended only for informational purposes and should thus be thought of as universal. As befitting its nature, it is presented without assurance regarding its prolonged validity or interim quality. Trademarks that are mentioned are done without written consent and can in no way be considered an endorsement from the trademark holder.

# Introduction and Overview as a Keto Vegan

Congratulations on downloading *The Vegan Keto Cookbook: Over 190 High-Fat Low-Carb Plant-Based Recipes to Shed and Heal You from the Inside Out*. By using the ketogenic diet with your vegan lifestyle, you are to receive many nutritional benefits from vegetables, fresh fruits, nuts, beans, whole grains, and soy products among others.

These are some of those benefits along with the positive effects it brings to your body:

- **Antioxidants**
  With this addition, you can protect your body against several types of cancer.
- **Carbohydrates**
  Your body tends to burn your muscle tissue if you don't eat plenty of carbs.
- **Vitamin C**
  This works as an antioxidant and helps your bruises heal faster and keeps your gums healthy.
- **Protein**
  As a vegan, lentils, nuts, peas, beans, and soy products provide this resource without health issues that can occur from red meats.
- **Fiber**
  The vegans experience better bowel movements with the increased high fiber in veggies and fruits.
- **Reduced Saturated Fats**
  Without the meats and dairy products, these levels lower immensely.
- **Magnesium**
  With the assistance of magnesium, calcium is better absorbed. It is found in dark leafy greens, seeds, and nuts.
- **Potassium**
  Acidity and water are balanced by potassium, which also leads to a reduction in cancer and cardiovascular diseases.

Some of the physical benefits can include body mass reduction, weight loss, higher energy levels, healthier skin, and many others. Supplements cannot replace a healthy diet plan according to experts.

Walnuts are a known source for "brainpower" food, but also, the others mentioned below are considered as superfoods:

- **Almonds**
  
  You can help to regulate your blood pressure as well as having a good source as an energy booster. Its antioxidant qualities are loaded with fiber and calcium. Just ¼ of a cup of almonds provides eight grams of vegan protein.

- **Blueberries**
  
  The high content of flavonoid antioxidants is what is accountable to have shown enhancement in memory, as well as general cognitive function and learning. The flavonoid categories to stock up on include maqui, acai, and cacao.

- **Chia Seeds**
  
  The rich omega-3 fatty acid content is abundant in the chia seeds, which helps enhance memory and protect against cognitive decline. You also receive a lower calorie boost.

- **Pumpkin Seeds**
  
  Pumpkin seeds provide a boost of zinc, which enhances your thinking and memory skills. Have some in seasonal soups, by the handful, or in a hearty salad.

- **Cranberries**
  
  The high concentration of ursolic acid helps protect your brain cells from degeneration and injury, possibly even reversing the damage. Choose the sun-dried ones without sugar and use a bit of fruit juice for sweetener, or have some of the berries fresh which is even more nutritious.

- **Strawberries**
  
  Not only are these berries loaded with antioxidants; they are a good source of vitamin C, along with 21% RDA of manganese. Strawberries also help fight cancer.

You will also want to use special spices while on the ketogenic diet plan. Save some money and know what is in your spices. Use these in your unique dishes as a vegan. It's vital to read each of the spice labels since many spice manufacturers include sugar.

You can flavor your foods using these spices to remain in ketosis:

- **High-Quality Salts**
  
  While you're on the ketogenic diet plan, your insulin levels decrease. Your kidneys naturally excrete higher sodium levels which, in turn, lower the

potassium/sodium ratio in your body. Increase the amount of sodium with one of these choices:

- Add 1/4 teaspoon of pink salt to your food or into a glass of water.
- Have a bowl of bone broth or use it in a keto recipe.
- Have a snack of pumpkin seeds or macadamia nuts.
- Add kelp or nori to your prepared foods.
- Slice celery and cucumber – both have natural sodium content.

- **Cinnamon**

Improve your insulin receptor activity by using cinnamon. Measure 1/2 teaspoon of cinnamon into a shake or any keto dessert. It is used extensively in many of the keto recipes.

- **Homemade Pumpkin Pie Spice:** Use this simple low-carb concoction for a healthier pastry dish.

> ### Pumpkin Pie Slice
>
> **Serving Yields:** 10.75 tsp. – 1 tsp. per serving
>
> **Macros:** 6.42 Calories| 0.8 g Net Carbs| 0.12 g Protein|0.09 g Total Fats
>
> **What You Need:**
> - Ground cinnamon – 2 tbsp.
> - Ground nutmeg - .5 tsp.
> - Ground ginger – 1 tbsp.
> - Allspice - .5 tsp
> - Cardamom - .25 tsp.
> - Ground cloves - .5 tsp. or .75 tsp. whole cloves

> **How to Prepare**:
> - Grind the cloves into powder using a spice grinder.
> - Combine all of the fixings in a mixing bowl until well combined
> - Store in a spice container to use any time the need arises.

- **Cayenne Pepper Hot Spices**
  Sprinkling dishes with Cayenne pepper increases your metabolism which helps burn away the fat. Cayenne is a stimulant for digestive enzymes and helps prevent stomach ulcers. Its anti-inflammatory elements make it a super choice for headaches, arthritis, or sore muscles. You can also receive a boost in your immunity as it clears away nasal congestion. Sprinkle your soups, stews, or chili.

- **Cumin Spice**
  This spice is an antioxidant and an excellent digestion reliever. It is a superior method to treat disorders such as bronchitis and asthma. It is also excellent for prediabetics or diabetes, and also for removing body fat. It's a great source for vitamins A and C as well as iron.

- **Turmeric Spices**
  Dating back to Ayurveda and Chinese medicine, this Asian orange herb has been known for its anti-inflammatory elements. It is so easy to add to your delicious veggies and smoothies. These are some of its benefits:
  - Excellent for weight management
  - Improves your digestion
  - Relieves arthritis
  - Helps control diabetes
  - Helps prevent Alzheimer's disease
  - Reduces your cholesterol levels

# Like what you're reading? Want to hear this as an audio book? Click here to get this book for FREE when you join Audible!!
https://adbl.co/2YmbdC8

- **Spicy and Sweet Cloves**

  Add cloves to hot tea for a spicy change. The germicidal and antiseptic ingredients in cloves help ease many types of pain, including:
  - The smell of cloves can help encourage mental creativity
  - Relief of digestive problems
  - Fights infections
  - Helps relieve arthritis pain
  - Helps relieve gum and tooth pain

- **Clove Oil**

  Clove oil is beneficial as an antiseptic to kill bacteria in fungal infections, itchy rashes, bruises, or burns.

- **Basil**

  You can use either dried or fresh basil to maximize the benefits. Its dark green color indicates that it also maintains an outstanding source of calcium, magnesium, and vitamin K (good for your bones). Basil helps cure some of these conditions:
  - Inflammatory bowel conditions
  - Allergies
  - Arthritis

- **Star Anise**

  This is one spice that is commonly used in the United States and also is applied in Indian, Chinese, Indonesian, and Malaysian dishes. Its licorice-like taste pairs with tomatoes. It can be found in powder and "star" form purchased in the whole form. Simply substitute Chinese Five Spice, common anise, or fennel seed. It is a super choice for its antibacterial, antifungal, and antioxidant qualities.

**Other Useful Spices**

- Cilantro
- Black Pepper
- Chili Powder

- **Fermented Foods and Probiotics**

   Enjoy a dish of yogurt. You can also include items such as kimchee, sauerkraut, pickles, coconut milk, or water kefir to benefit your digestive system. Fermented foods help restore the "good" bacteria in your gut. The natural acids help stabilize your blood sugar levels as well as the enzymes, probiotics, and other bioactive nutrients help support ketosis.

- **Healthy Fats**

   To achieve success in the ketogenic diet, you need fats. Fats are an essential part of your diet, but it is essential to know which ones are beneficial to your health and the ones that can be dangerous. Monounsaturated and Saturated Fats include avocado, coconut oil, and macadamia nuts are some of the recommended categories. These products can be incorporated into your meals using various recipes.

   Use non-hydrogenated lards or coconut oil. Less oxidation occurs in the oil because they have higher smoke points than other oils. These are some of those:

   - Avocado
   - Coconut Oil
   - Red Palm Oil
   - Sesame, avocado, and coconut oil
   - Flaxseed oil
   - Coconut flakes
   - Macadamia nuts
   - Macadamia Oil: One of the benefits of this oil is that it has a high smoke point. It carries a mild flavor which is a super alternative to olive oil in mayonnaise.
   - Olives

- **Extra-Virgin Olive Oil (EVOO)**

Olive oil is one of the oldest edible oils in existence, with culinary uses dating back to at least 1000 B.C. and even more in the distance was the oil used for anointing priests and kings. It's versatile, delicious, and good for your health.

Research shows that olive oil helps prevent cardiovascular disease by protecting the integrity of your vascular system and lowering LDL "bad" cholesterol. Furthermore, after new research, extra-virgin olive oil also improves the gut microbiome by increasing the growth of probiotic Bifidobacterium strains.

Monounsaturated fats, like the ones in olive oil, are also linked with better blood sugar regulation, lower fasting glucose, and reducing inflammation throughout the body. Research further indicates that extra-virgin olive oil resists oxidation during the heating process much better than many other cooking oils, which makes it have a smoke point as high as 410°F.

## Make Use of Low-Carb Substitutions

### Chia Seeds

The seeds can absorb up to 11 times its weight in liquid. Be sure to add plenty of water and soak them for at least five minutes before using in your keto recipes. Otherwise, you will have some uncomfortable digestion after eating them. As always, be sure to remain hydrated.

### Limes and Lemons

Your blood sugar levels naturally drop with these citric additions, and also, signal a boost in your liver function. Use them with a salad, in green juices, or with cooked with meats or veggies. The following are the benefits of lime and lemon:

- Excellent for weight loss
- Balances pH
- Blood purifier
- Relieves respiratory infections
- Reduces fever
- Reduces toothache pain
- Boosts your immune system
- Decreases wrinkles and blemishes
- Flushes out the unwanted, unhealthy materials

### Apple Cider Vinegar

You can add just one to two tablespoons of vinegar to an 8-ounce glass of water to help the process, or take a shot of vinegar solo. These are just a few ways this helps your progress:

- Helps you to drop the pounds
- Helps with sore muscles
- Improves your digestion tract
- Excellent for detoxification
- A good energy booster
- Reduces cholesterol
- Controls sugar intake/aids in diabetes
- Strengthens your immune system
- Balances your inner body system and functions

## Select Keto-Friendly Sweeteners

### Stevia Drops

Stevia Drops offer delicious flavors including hazelnut, vanilla, English toffee, and chocolate. Enjoy making a satisfying cup of sweetened coffee or other healthy drinks. Some individuals think the drops are too bitter, so use only three drops to equal one teaspoon of sugar.

### Pyure's Organic All-Purpose Blend

Pyure's Organic All-Purpose Blend is considered as the best all-around sweetener with less of a bitter after-taste versus a stevia-based product. The blend of stevia and erythritol is an excellent alternative to baking, sweetening desserts, and various cooking needs.

The substitution ratio is one teaspoon of sugar for each one-third teaspoon of Pyure. Just add the blend slowly and adjust to your taste. You can always add a bit more. If you need powdered sugar, grind the sweetener in a NutriBullet or high-speed blender until it maintains a dry consistency.

### Xylitol

This is excellent for sweetening your barbecue sauce and teriyaki; it tastes just like sugar! The natural occurring sugar alcohol has the Glycemic index (GI) standing of 13. If you have tried others and weren't satisfied, this might be for you.

Xylitol also helps keep your mouth bacteria in check and is commonly found in chewing gum. However, don't use it often in large amounts since it can cause diarrhea - making chewing gum a laxative if used in large quantities.

*Note:* If you have a puppy in the house, be sure to use caution since it is toxic to dogs - even small amounts.

### Swerve Granular Sweetener

Swerve is also an excellent choice as a blend. It's made of non-digestible carbs sourced from starchy root veggies and select fruits. Start with 3/4 of a teaspoon for every one of sugar. Increase the portion to your taste.

Swerve also has its own confectioner's powdered sugar for your baking needs. Unfortunately, it's more expensive (about twice the price) than other products such as the Pyure.

### Pancake Syrup

Lakanto's Maple-Flavored Syrup is an exceptional choice for pancake syrup since it is "monk fruit" and erythritol-based.

### Brown Sugar Option

Golden Monk Fruit Sweetener is an excellent choice for brown sugar. The name "monk fruit" came from the Buddhist monks over 1,000 years ago and is considered a cooling agent. It may not agree with your digestive system, so use it frugally if using in baked goods.

## Ketogenic Vegetable Choices

Each of these has the Net Carbs listed per 100 grams or 1/2 cup:

Alfalfa Seeds – Sprouted - 0.2

Arugula – 2.05
Asparagus – 1.78
Bamboo shoots: 3
Beans – Green snap – 3.6
Beet greens – 0.63
Bell pepper
Broccoli – 4.04
Cabbage – Savoy – 3
Carrots – 6.78
Carrots – baby – 5.34
Cauliflower – 2.97
Celery – 1.37
Chard – 2.14
Chicory greens – 0.7
Chives – 1.85
Coriander – Cilantro Leaves – 0.87
Cucumber with Peel – 3.13
Eggplant – 2.88
Garlic – 30.96
Ginger root – 15.77
Kale – 5.15
Leeks – bulb (+) lower leaf – 12.35
Lemongrass – citronella 25.31
Lettuce – red leaf – 1.36
Lettuce – crisp-head types ex. iceberg 1.77
Mushrooms brown – 3.7
Mustard Greens – 1.47
Onions – yellow – 7.64
Onions – scallions or spring – 4.74
Onions – sweet – 6.65
Peppers – banana – 1.95
Peppers – red hot chili – 7.31
Peppers – jalapeno – 3.7
Peppers – sweet – green – 2.94
Peppers – sweet – red – 3.93
Peppers – sweet – yellow – 5.42
Portabella Mushrooms – 2.57
Pumpkin – 6
Radishes – 1.8
Seaweed – kelp – 8.27
Seaweed – spirulina - 2.02

Shiitake mushrooms – 4.29
Spinach – 1.43
Squash – crookneck - summer – 2.64
Squash - Zucchini – 2.11
Squash – winter – acorn – 8.92
Tomatoes – 2.69
Turnips – 4.63
Turnip Greens – 3.93
White Mushrooms – 2.26

You may want to consider these for your dieting needs as well:
- 
- Parsnips
- Squash
- Peas
- Zucchini

## Get Your Nutrients from Veggies

### Calcium

Strong bones, muscle contraction, and proper blood clotting are all elements involved with calcium. Use these sources to add to your calcium counts:
- Leafy greens such as broccoli
- Dairy and non-dairy milk – unsweetened and zero carbs

You may need to supplement with calcium supplements including Vitamin D which is necessary for absorption. Both women and men should consume approximately 1000 mg — daily of calcium.

### Vitamin D

Vitamin D supplies nutrients and hormones in your body. You cannot always get enough from your food, but you can go outside and take in some fresh air and sunshine for your portion. Use caution from over-exposure and the risks of skin cancer. The D vitamin also helps your body absorb magnesium, calcium, and other essential minerals to maintain your muscle growth and bone density. If yours is low, you are like about 1/3 of all Americans. Supplement the same by adding 400 IU per day as recommended, and add mushrooms to your diet plan.

**Beta Carotene**

Many foods contain beta carotene. However, a lot of them are higher in carbs, so the typically vegan keto dieter may not be getting a sufficient supply. Also, it should be noted that high levels of vitamin A in the body are toxic, so be careful if you are using supplements or try to get your beta carotene from whole food sources. Below is a list of several keto friendly foods that contain beta carotene:

- Asparagus
- Broccoli
- Collard Greens
- Dandelion Greens
- Kale
- Onions
- Peppers
- Spinach
- Pumpkin

Note: The brighter and more vibrant the yellow-orange color, the higher the levels of beta carotene; the chlorophyll hides the yellow-orange in leafy greens.

**Chlorella**

The green algae superfood is good for fighting off fatigue. It contains Chlorella Growth Factor – a nutrient containing DNA and RNA to help increase energy transport between your cells. You can purchase the supplement in powder form, tablets, or capsules. Mix it with water, a smoothie, or other drinks and have one daily.

## Spirulina

The blue-green algae are similar to chlorella and contain all the amino acids your body requires which makes it a complete protein. It also contains magnesium, iron, potassium, and other beneficial nutrients. It has superb antioxidant properties. The medication has shown positive results with individuals who suffer from cholesterol and high blood pressure. It raises the HDL (good cholesterol) and, at the same time, lowers the LDL (bad cholesterol). You can purchase in capsule form or in powder to mix in water or with a tasty smoothie.

## Select Fresh Fruits

This collection of keto fruits for each 1/2 cup serving – listed in grams per serving:

- 
- Apples – no skin - boiled – 13.6
- Apricots 7.5
- Bananas 23.4
- Blackberries – 23.1
- Blueberries – 22.1
- Cantaloupe - 6
- Kiwi – 14.2
- Oranges – 11.7
- Peaches – 11.6
- Pears – 19.2
- Pineapple – 11
- Plums – 16.3
- Kiwi - 15
- Watermelon 7.1

These are a few more that are acceptable for the Keto diet plan:

- 
- Lemon juice
- Lime juice
- Strawberries
- Casaba Melon
- Green olives
- Avocados
- Coconut
- Rhubarb
- Black Olives
- Carambola aka Starfruit
- Gooseberries
- Acerola aka West Indian Cherry
- Oheloberries
- Boysenberries
- Grapefruit

*Note:* Values for the fruits and vegetables are rough estimates for general information. Each of the recipes using these items (in this book) has values calculated in the totals.

Let's see how all of these delicious recipes will blend with your chosen meals as you adjust to a new lifestyle. Please enjoy!

# Chapter 1: Morning and Brunch Specialties

## Begin A Ketogenic Routine

Start each morning (or your waking time) with a large glass of water. You can also add a supplement with MCT oil. Try this for maximum "get up and go" technique:

## Bulletproof Coffee

**Nutritional Counts:** Net Carbs: -0- g | Totals Fat: 51 g

**Ingredients:**

- MCT oil powder - 2 tbsp.
- Canned coconut milk - 2 tbsp.
- Hot coffee – 1.5 cups

**Preparation Method:**

- Pour the hot coffee into your blender.

- Add the powder and milk. Blend until creamy and frothy.
- Enjoy served in a large mug at home or on-the-go.

## Bulletproof Tea

**Nutritional Counts:** Net Carbs: 1 g| Total Fats: 17 g

**Ingredients:**

- Strong tea – 10 oz.
- Coconut or MCT oil – 1 tbsp.
- Canned coconut milk – 1 tbsp.
- Ground cinnamon - .125 tsp.
- Optional: Collagen peptides – 1 scoop

**Preparation Method:**

- Combine all of the fixings in a tall mug.
- Blend until frothy.

## Pancake Time

### Cinnamon Roll Pancakes

**Serving Yields**: 3

**Nutritional Counts**: Net Carbs: 0.5 g| Fat: 7 g

**Ingredients:**

- Rolled oats or quinoa flakes – 1 cup
- Milk of choice - .25 to .5 cup
- Unsweetened applesauce or sub. pumpkin - banana or sweet potato - .5 cup
- Cinnamon – 1 tsp.
- Apple cider vinegar or sub with lemon or lime juice – 1 tbsp.
- Baking powder – 1 tsp.
- Sticky sweetener of choice – 1 tbsp.
- Vanilla – 1 tsp.

**For Cinnamon Roll Glaze:**

- Coconut butter – 1-2 tbsp.

- Cinnamon – 1 tsp.
- Milk of choice – 1 tbsp.

**Preparation Method:**

- In a high-speed blender, such as a NutriBullet, mix in each of your fixings and pulse until thoroughly combined and a thick batter remains.
- Allow the batter to rest for 5-10 minutes, allowing the coconut flour/rolled oats to thicken. If it isn't thin enough, just continue adding milk a little at a time.
- Preheat a greased/oiled pan over low-med temperature setting.
- Pour scant 1/4 cup portions of batter on the hot pan. Cover the pan and cook for two to three minutes, until bubbles form on the edges. Then, just flip them over. Continue cooking until all the batter is used up.
- Once pancakes are cooked, prepare your sticky cinnamon roll glaze. Melt your coconut butter and add the cinnamon. Thin out with milk and drizzle over the top.

## Coconut Pancakes

**Serving Yields**: 2

**Nutritional Counts**: Net Carbs: 1 g| Fat: 7 g

**Ingredients:**

- Water – 1 cup
- Protein powder – 1 oz.
- Coconut flour - .25 cup
- Coconut oil - 1 tbsp.
- Baking powder – 1 tsp.

- Vanilla – 1 tsp.
- Psyllium husk powder – 2 tbsp. – to soak in .5 cup water

**Preparation Method**

- In a mixing bowl; combine the dry components.
- Combine the vanilla and coconut oil into the soaked psyllium husk.
- Add water to the dry fixings, and mix it well.
- Using the medium heat setting, spoon the batter into a warm skillet.
- Cook for five minutes and flip. Continue cooking for 5 more minutes. Continue the process until you have your meal ready.
- Serve and enjoy with your favorite toppings. Just be sure to add the extra carbs and fats.
- Special Tip: The psyllium husk has many health benefits including lowering your cholesterol and relieving constipation.

## Crispy Flaxseed Waffles

**Serving Yields**: 4

**Nutritional Counts**: Net Carbs: 3 g| Fat: 42 g

**Ingredients:**

- Roughly ground golden flaxseed – 2 cups
- Gluten-free baking powder – 1 tbsp.
- Sea salt – 1 tsp.
- Finely ground flaxseed – 5 tbsp. (+) 15 tbsp. warm water.
- Water - .5 cup
- Avocado oil or extra-virgin olive oil or melted coconut oil - .33 cup
- Fresh herbs – 1 tbsp. (if making savory) or 2 tsp. ground cinnamon

**Preparation Method:**

- Arrange the waffle maker on the countertop and warm it up using the medium heat setting for crispy waffles.

- Combine the sea salt with the flaxseed and baking powder in a big mixing container. Mix well and set to the side for now.

- Pour the 15 tbsp. of warm water into the 5 tbsp. of ground flaxseed (replaces the regular egg) with the .5 cup of water. Let it sit for 5 minutes and add the oil to the jug of a high-powered blender. Blend using the high setting until it is foamy or about 30 seconds.

- Pour the liquid mixture into the bowl with the flaxseed mixture. Stir well until barely incorporated. The mixture will be very fluffy. Once combined, let it sit for about three minutes.

- Add in your fresh herbs or stir in the ground cinnamon.

- Divide mixture into 4 servings. Scoop each; one at a time, onto the preheated waffle maker and close the top. Cook until it beeps, and continue cooking with remaining batter.

- Eat immediately or freeze in an air-tight container for a couple of weeks. Can be frozen and then toasted for a quick breakfast, lunch or dinner.

- *Note:* You can also use 10 teaspoons of finely ground chia seed and 15 tablespoons warm water (step 3). You can also garnish with some fresh strawberries.

## Flaxseed Pancakes

**Serving Yields**: 1

**Nutritional Counts**: Net Carbs: 2.2 g| Fat: 27.1 g

### Ingredients:

- Water - 3 tbsp.
- Flaxseeds – divided - 2 tbsp.
- Salt – 1 pinch
- Baking powder - .25 tsp.
- Coconut oil – 1.5 tbsp.
- Vanilla flavor vegan powder - .5 of a scoop

### Preparation Method:

- Combine the water with half (1 tbsp.) of the seeds. Stir in the oil. Set aside for a minute.
- Whisk the baking powder, rest of the seeds, salt, and protein powder in a separate container.
- Stir the fixings together and warm up a skillet (medium heat).
- Add the batter to the prepared pan. Cook for five minutes on the first side. Gently turn the pancake and continue cooking two more minutes. Do the same with the rest of the batter.

# Scallion Pancakes

**Serving Yields**: 4

**Nutritional Counts**: Net Carbs: 4.7 g| Fat: 16.1 g

**Ingredients:**

- Scallions – white and green parts – sliced - 3
- Psyllium husk powder – 2 tbsp.
- Coconut flour - .5 cup
- Salt - .25 tsp.
- Garlic powder - .5 tsp.
- Sesame oil - .25 cup
- Warm water – 1 cup

**Ingredients for the Sauce:**

- Minced clove of garlic – 1
- Rice wine vinegar – 1 tsp.
- Water -1 tbsp.
- Sesame oil – 1 tsp.
- Tamari - 1 tbsp.
- Chili flakes – to taste

**Preparation Method:**

- Mix the scallions, water, garlic, and salt in a container and set aside for about five minutes.

- In another dish, whisk the husk powder and flour.

- Combine the fixings to form a dough. Prepare into four portions and flatten using your hands.

- Warm up the oil in a skillet. Place a dough round in the hot, flattening with the spatula. Cook for five minutes on each side and continue with the remainder of the dough sections.

- Combine the sauce components and serve with the tasty scallion pancakes.

## Other Delicious Choices

### Almonds and Chips Breakfast Cereal

**Serving Yields:** 1

**Nutritional Counts:** Net Carbs: 3 g| Fat: 27 g

Ingredients:

- Coconut milk - .25 cup
- Hemp hearts – 3 tbsp.
- Shredded coconut - .5 tbsp.
- Chocolate chips - .5 tbsp.
- Chopped almonds - .5 tbsp.
- Liquid stevia – 1 drop

**Preparation Method:**

- Combine the fixings in a jar or bowl with a lid.
- Stir well and place in the fridge for a minimum of 4 hrs. (overnight is better).
- Enjoy cold or warm.

# Avocado – Carrot and Tahini Breakfast Bowl

**Serving Yields: 1**

**Nutritional Counts:** Net Carbs: 5.5 g| Fat: 52 g

**Ingredients:**

- Carrot - 1
- Haas avocado - 1
- Tahini – 2 tbsp.

**for the SAUCE:**

- Grated ginger – 1 tsp.
- Salt - .25 tsp.
- Lemon juice - .25 cup
- Olive oil - .25 cup
- Poppy seeds – 1 tbsp.

**Preparation Method:**

- Slice the avocado in half and remove the pit. Shred the carrot. Set aside.
- Whisk the sauce fixings. Mix the shredded carrot with 2 tbsp. of the sauce (save some for later).
- Stuff the carrots into the avocado wells and sprinkle with the tahini.
- Have a relaxing breakfast before you start your day.

# Bagel Thins for Breakfast

**Serving Yields**: 6

**Nutritional Counts**: Net Carbs: -0- g| Fat: 16.4 g

## Ingredients:

- Ground flax seed - .5 cup
- Tahini - .5 cup
- Psyllium husks - .25 cup
- Water – 1 cup
- Baking powder – 1 tsp.
- Salt – 1 pinch or add up to 1 tsp if using unsalted tahini)
- Optional - sesame seeds for garnish

## Preparation Method:

- Warm up the oven to 375°F.

- Add the following to a mixing bowl: Psyllium husk, ground flax seeds, baking powder, and salt. Whisk until thoroughly combined. Pour in the water to the tahini, and whisk until combined.
- Stir the dry ingredients into the wet, and then knead to form the dough. It's important that everything is kneaded thoroughly and that the dough is incorporated.
- Form patties by hand that are about 4-inches in diameter, and 1/4-inch thick. Lay on your baking tray and cut a small circle from the middle of each round.
- You can also use a doughnut pan for this step, which makes everything so much easier!

## Berry and Nut Cereal

**Serving Yields:** 1

**Nutritional Counts:** Net Carbs: 2.96 g| Fat: 32.59 g

### Ingredients:

- Chopped strawberries - 2
- Blueberries - 2 tbsp.
- Walnuts - 2 tbsp.
- Pecans - 3 tbsp.
- Almonds - 3 tbsp.
- Sweetener to taste - 3 tbsp.
- For Serving: Coconut milk

### Preparation Method:

- Chop the almonds, pecans, and walnuts.
- Combine each of the fixings into one mixing container (omit the milk).
- Slowly add the milk last.

# Blueberry Breakfast Cake – Flourless and Gluten-Free

**Serving Yields**: 12

**Nutritional Counts**: Net Carbs: 3 g| Fat: 11 g

**Ingredients:**

- Rolled oats - gluten-free ground into a flour – 2 cups
- Baking powder – 1 tbsp.
- Coconut palm sugar - .5 cup or any granulated sweetener of choice
- Sea salt – 1 pinch
- Milk of choice – 1 cup
- Flax egg – 1 (ground chia (+) 3 tbsp. water or 1 tbsp. of ground flax )
- Vanilla extract – 1 tsp.
- Smooth almond butter or any nut/seed butter of choice – 6 tbsp.
- Blueberries - .25 to .5 cup

**Preparation Method:**

- Warm up the oven to reach 350°F.
- Cover a square pan or loaf pan using a sheet of parchment paper and place to the side for now.
- In a large container, add your dry fixings and stir well.
- In another container, beat the eggs well. Stir in the melted coconut oil, unsweetened applesauce and sticky sweetener of choice and mix very well.
- Mix each of the fixings in a high-speed blender until a smooth batter remains. Fold in the blueberries.

- Pour your blueberry breakfast cake batter in the lined pan and bake for 35-40 minutes. Check for doneness using a toothpick. It is done when it comes out clean from the center. Cool in the pan for about ten minutes.
- Once the cake is cooled, prepare your frosting before topping the cake and cutting into slices.

## Bran Muffins – Gluten-Free

**Serving Yields**: 6

**Nutritional Counts**: Net Carbs: 1 g| Fat: 4 g

**Ingredients:**

- Ground flax - .5 cup
- Flax or chia eggs - 2
- Oat fiber - .25 cup
- Coconut flour – 2 tbsp.

- Baking soda - .25 tsp.
- Cinnamon - 1 tsp.
- Baking powder - .5 tsp
- Water - .25 cup
- Lakanto Monk Fruit Sweetener – or another granulated option - .5 cup or another granulated sweetener of choice
- Vanilla extract - .25 tsp.

**Preparation Method:**

- Prepare the flax/chia eggs using 6 tbsp. of water and ground chia or 2 tbsp. of ground flax. Set aside.
- Warm up the oven to reach 350°F. Spritz muffin tins with some non-stick cooking spray, and set aside.
- Combine the oat fiber, 1/2 cup flax, sweetener, coconut flour, cinnamon, baking soda, and baking powder in a large mixing bowl. Mix well with a fork.
- Pour in the water, vanilla extract, and flax/chia eggs. Mix well. Spoon into the prepared muffin tins.
- Bake for 35 minutes.

## Breakfast Quiche

**Serving Yields:** 5

**Nutritional Counts:** Net Carbs: 8.6 g| Fat: 37.7 g

**Ingredients:**

- Water – 3 tbsp.
- Olive oil – 2 tbsp.

- Chopped zucchini – 1.5 cups
- Salt - .5 tsp.
- Turmeric - .25 tsp.
- Black pepper – to taste
- Firm tofu – 14 oz.
- Low-carb vegan-friendly crust - 1

**Preparation Method:**

- Program the oven setting to 350°F.
- Warm up the oil in a skillet and slowly cook the zucchini.
- Mix the turmeric, pepper, salt, tofu, and water until you reach a thick consistency.
- Fold in the zucchini and stir well, adding the mixture to the crust.
- Prepare for 30 minutes until the ingredients are set.
- Relax and enjoy a slice of heaven!

## Cinnamon Roll Muffins

**Serving Yields**: 20

**Nutritional Counts**: Net Carbs: -0- g| Fat: 9 g

**Ingredients:**

- Almond flour - .5 cup
- Vanilla protein powder 2 scoops (32-34 g per scoop)
- Baking powder – 1 tsp.
- Cinnamon – 1 tbsp.

- Nut or seed butter of choice almond, peanut, or sunflower seed butter, etc. - .5 cup

- Pumpkin puree can sub for unsweetened applesauce, mashed banana or mashed cooked sweet potato - .5 cup

- Coconut oil - .5 cup

**for the glaze:**

- Coconut butter - .25 cup

- Milk of choice - .25 cup

- Granulated sweetener of choice – 1 tbsp.

- Lemon juice – 2 tsp.

**Preparation Method:**

- Heat up the oven temperature to reach 350°F.

- Line a 12-count muffin tin with paper liners and set aside. This can also be made using a mini muffin tin.

- In a large mixing container, mix your dry ingredients and mix well. Add your wet fixings. Combine well until fully incorporated.

- Evenly distribute the cinnamon roll muffin batter evenly in the muffin liners.

- Bake for 10-15 minutes, checking around the 10-minute mark by inserting a skewer in the center and seeing if it comes out clean. If it does, muffins are done. Allow cooling in pan for 5 minutes, before transferring to a wire rack to cool completely.

- Once cooled, prepare your cinnamon roll glaze by combining all ingredients and mixing until combined. Drizzle over the muffin tops and allow to firm up.

- The muffins should be kept refrigerated for optimum freshness. They can be kept at room temperature, in a covered container, but must be eaten within 2 days. To freeze muffins, wrap each serving individually.

## Macadamia Breakfast Bars

**Serving Yields:** 5

**Nutritional Counts**: Net Carbs: 9 g| Fat: 42 g

### Ingredients:

- Coconut oil - .25 cup
- Crushed Macadamia nuts – 2.1 oz.
- Almond butter - .5 cup
- Unsweetened shredded coconut – 6 tbsp.
- Stevia drops - 20

### Preparation Method:

- Combine the fixings in a mixing container. Pour it into a parchment paper-lined baking dish.
- Place in the refrigerator overnight for the best results.

## Maple Walnut Breakfast Cereal

**Serving Yields:** 1

**Nutritional Counts:** Net Carbs: 2.47 g| Fat: 6.48 g

### Ingredients:

- Chopped walnuts – 1 tbsp.
- Hemp hearts – 3 tbsp.

- Sugar-free maple syrup - .5 tbsp.
- Almond milk – 3 tbsp.
- Cinnamon - .5 tsp.
- Chia seeds – 1 tsp.

**Preparation Method:**

- Combine the fixings in a jar or bowl.
- Mix well and place in the fridge for at least four hours. Overnight is best.
- Serve either cold or warm.

## Minty Eggplant Hash Browns

**Serving Yields:** 8

**Nutritional Counts:** Net Carbs: 5.26 g| Fat: 6.4 g

**Ingredients:**

- Coconut oil – 2 tbsp.
- Red bell peppers - 2
- Eggplant - 1
- Garlic cloves - 4
- Red onion - 1
- Fresh mint leaves - .25 cup
- Toasted slivered almonds - .25 cup
- Sundried tomatoes in oil - .5 cup
- Ground cayenne pepper - .25 tsp.

- Ground coriander - .5 tsp.
- Ground cinnamon - .5 tsp.
- Salt and Pepper – to your liking

**Preparation Method:**

- Prep the Veggies: Peel and cube the eggplant, mince the garlic cloves, and dice the peppers and onions.
- Warm up the oil in a skillet. Sear the peppers and eggplant for 3 minutes – stir occasionally. Toss in the onion and garlic. Continue to saute for two additional minutes. Stir in the rest of the fixings.
- Toss well and remove from the flame. Transfer to a serving platter and enjoy with your family and friends.

## Muesli in the Raw

**Serving Yields:** 20

**Nutritional Counts:** Net Carbs: 4.2 g| Fat: 26 g

**Ingredients:**

- Unsweetened shredded coconut – 2 cups
- Ground linseed – 1 cup
- Sesame seeds – 1 cup
- Pumpkin seeds – 1 cup
- Pieces of walnuts – 1 cup
- Chopped almonds – 1 cup
- Sunflower seeds – 1 cup

**Preparation Method:**

- Mix all of the fixings and seal in an airtight jar.
- When ready to serve; just add some coconut cream and enjoy!
- Note: Be sure to count the carbs for each serving to remain in ketosis.

## Peanut Butter Breakfast Cereal

**Serving Yields:** 1

**Nutrition Counts:** Net Carbs: 3 g| Fat: 27 g

**Ingredients:**

- Hemp hearts – 3 tbsp.
- Peanut butter – 1 tbsp.
- Chia seeds – 1 tsp.
- Almond milk – 3 tbsp.
- Liquid stevia – 1 drop

**Preparation Method:**

- Combine and mix the ingredients well in a bowl or mason jar.
- Store the chosen container in the refrigerator overnight for the best results or for a minimum of four hours.
- Serve hot or cold.

## Psyllium Breakfast Mix

**Serving Yields:** 23

**Nutritional Counts**: Net Carbs: 2.3 g| Fat: 3.8 g

**Ingredients:**

- Hemp seeds – 7 tbsp.
- Ground flaxseed - 5 tbsp.
- Psyllium husk - 2 tbsp.
- Ground sesame -2 tbsp.
- Dark unsweetened cocoa - 2 tbsp.
- Unsweetened coconut flakes - 5 tbsp.

**Preparation Method:**

- Combine all of the components in a mason jar.
- Seal the jar and shake well.
- Serve with some black coffee or water.

## Pumpkin Pie Breakfast Cereal

**Serving Yields**: 1

**Nutritional Counts:** Net Carbs: 3 g| Fat: 27 g

**Ingredients:**

- Pumpkin puree – 1 tbsp.
- Pumpkin pie spice - .5 tsp.
- Hemp hearts - 3 tbsp.
- Chia seeds – 1 tsp.

- Almond milk - 3 tbsp.
- Liquid stevia – 2 drops

**Preparation Method:**
- Combine all of the fixings in a mason jar.
- Mix well and refrigerate overnight for the best results.
- Enjoy in the morning – either hot or cold.

## Scrambled Tofu

**Serving Yields:** 4
**Nutritional Counts**: Net Carbs: 9.7 g| Fat: 11.5 g

**Ingredients:**
- Olive oil – 1 tbsp.
- Diced tomatoes - 1 can - 14.5 oz.
- Chopped green onions – 1 bunch
- Firm silken tofu - 1 pkg. - 12 oz.

**Optional Fixings:**
- Pepper and salt
- Ground turmeric
- Optional: Vegan cheese - .5 cup

**Preparation Method:**
- Chop and saute the onions. Using medium heat, heat up oil in a skillet, and slowly cook the onions until translucent.
- Blend in the tomatoes along with the juices and the mashed tofu.
- Add the turmeric, pepper, and salt for flavoring and heat.
- Garnish as desired.

## Seed and Nut-Packed Bread

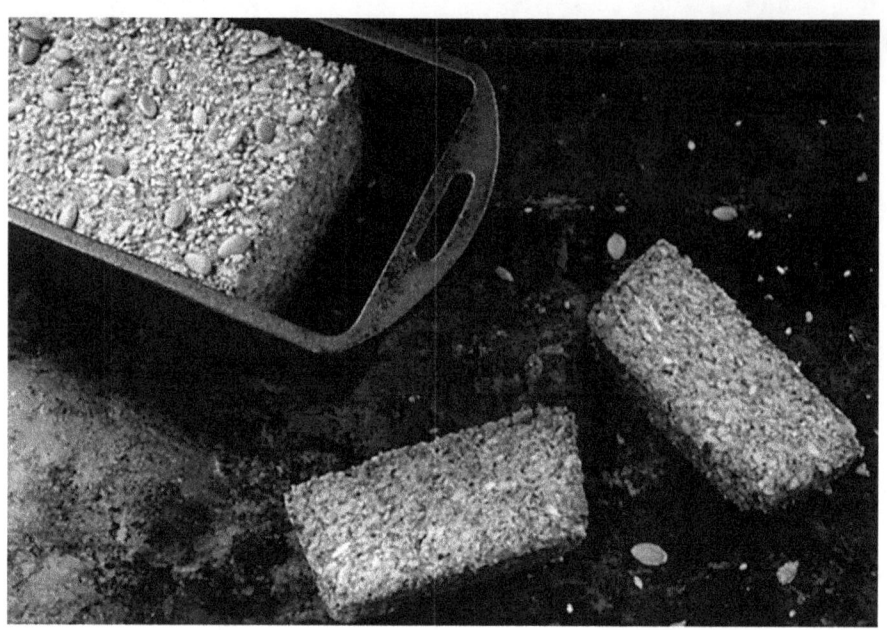

**Serving Yields**: 8

**Nutritional Counts:** Net Carbs: 4 g| Fat: 19 g

**Ingredients:**

- Psyllium husk powder – 3 tbsp.
- Sunflower seeds - .5 cup
- Pumpkin seeds - .5 cup
- Chia seeds – 2 tbsp.
- Onion powder – 1 tsp.
- Water - .33 cup
- Flaxseed meal - .33 cup
- Coconut oil - .33 cup
- Salt – 1 tsp.
- Almond slices - .33 cup

**Preparation Method:**

- Prepare a baking tin with a sheet of parchment paper.
- Warm up the oven to reach 350°F.
- Combine the dry fixings in a mixing dish.
- Stir in the oil until the mixture is crumbly.
- Slowly add the water until it has a right dough consistency.
- Spread it out in the pan. Arrange the pan in the preheated oven.
- Bake for 15 minutes. Take it out and gently slice it into squares.
- Put the pan back in the oven. Bake for 30 additional minutes.

## Vanilla and Turmeric Breakfast Cereal

**Serving Yields:** 1

**Nutritional Counts:** Net Carbs: 3 g| Fat: 27 g

**Ingredients:**

- Coconut milk - .25 cup
- Chia seeds – 1 tsp.
- Hemp hearts – 3 tbsp.
- Liquid stevia – 2 drops
- Vanilla extract - .5 tsp.
- Turmeric powder - .5 tsp.

**Preparation Method:**

- Mix together all of the fixings. Pour into a covered bowl or jar.
- Refrigerate for at least four hours, but it's best if chilled overnight.
- Serve either warm or cold.

## Oatmeal and Porridge Favorites

### Berries and Hemp Seeds

**Serving Yields**: 1

**Nutritional Counts**: Net Carbs: 3.10 g| Fat: 19.13 g

**Ingredients:**

- Boiling water - .5 cup
- Hemp hearts – 2 tbsp.
- Chia seeds – 1 tbsp.
- Unsweetened coconut flakes – 2 tbsp.
- For the Garnish: Stevia, cinnamon, and frozen berries – to your liking

**Preparation Method:**

- Mix all of the fixings in a medium mixing container. Pour in the water. Stir well.
- Let it steep for about 5 minutes and serve.

### Blueberry Porridge

**Serving Yields:** 2

**Nutritional Counts**: Net Carbs: 8 g| Fat: 34 g

**Ingredients:**

- Almond milk – 1 cup
- Coconut flour - .25 cup
- Ground flaxseed - .25 cup
- Vanilla extract – 1 tsp.
- Cinnamon – 1 tsp.
- Liquid stevia – 10 drops
- Salt - 1 pinch

**Preparation Method:**

- Warm up the milk on the stovetop using the low heat setting. Whisk in the cinnamon, salt, flaxseed, and flour.

- At the time it begins bubbling, stir in the stevia and vanilla. Once it starts thickening, remove the porridge from the burner.
- Serve and enjoy with a topping of blueberries, pumpkin seeds, and shaved coconut.

## Fudge Oatmeal

**Serving Yields**: 2

**Nutritional Counts**: Net Carbs: 4.5 g| Fat: 39.4 g

**Ingredients:**

- Hemp hearts - .5 cup
- Full-fat coconut milk - .33 cup
- Sunflower butter - 1 tbsp.
- Chia seeds - 1 tbsp.
- Cacao powder – 2 tbsp.
- Liquid stevia – 3 drops
- Himalayan rock salt – finely ground – 1 pinch
- Vanilla extract - .5 tsp.

**Preparation Method:**

- Mix all of the fixings in a mason jar and shake well.
- Place in the fridge overnight for the tastiest results.

# Overnight Oat Options

## Alternative #1: Vanilla Oats: The Base

**Serving Yields**: 2

**Nutritional Counts**: Net Carbs: 2.9 g| Fat: 34.7 g

**Ingredients:**

- Full-fat coconut milk - .33 cup (+) more next day
- Hemp hearts - .5 cup
- Chia seeds – 1 tbsp.
- Liquid stevia – 3-4 drops
- Vanilla extract - .5 tsp.
- Himalayan rock salt – finely ground – A pinch

**Ingredients for optional toppings:**

- Whole raspberries - 6
- Whole almonds - 12

**Preparation Method:**

- Combine all of the fixings into a container (12 oz. minimum) with a top.
- Stir well and cover in the refrigerator 8 hours to overnight.
- In the morning, add the milk if you like it and enjoy it.

## Alternative #2: Pumpkin Spice Latte Overnight Oats

**Serving Yields**: 2

**Nutritional Counts**: Net Carbs: 9.4 g| Fat: 26.7 g

**Ingredients:**

- Canned pumpkin puree – 2 tbsp.
- Pumpkin spice or 3/8 tsp. –
    - Ground cinnamon - .5 tsp.
    - Ground cloves - .125 tsp.
    - Ground nutmeg - .25 tsp.
- 1 main recipe (Vanilla Oats: The Base: Variation 1)

*Omit*: 1/3 cup of the coconut milk and replace it with 1/3 cup of the brewed coffee.

**Optional Toppings:**

- Ground cinnamon
- Pecans

## Alternative #3: Fudge Overnight Oats

**Serving Yields**: 2

**Nutritional Counts**: Net Carbs: 4.5 g| Fat: 39.4 g

**Additional Ingredients:**

- 1 recipe above (Vanilla Oats: The Base: Variation 1)
- Cacao powder – 2 tbsp.
- Sunflower butter – 1 tbsp.

**Optional Toppings**

- Cacao Nibs
- Shredded unsweetened coconut
- Strawberries

## Porridge Options

### Delicious Plain Porridge

**Serving Yields**: 1

**Nutritional Counts:** Net Carbs: 5.78 g | Fat: 13.1 g

**Ingredients:**

- Golden flaxseed meal – 3 tbsp.
- Coconut flour – 2 tbsp.
- Vanilla protein powder – vegan – 2 tbsp.
- Unsweetened almond milk – 1.5 cup
- Powdered erythritol – to your liking

**Preparation Method:**

- Combine the flaxseed meal, flour, and protein powder in a bowl.
- Pour the milk into a saucepan using the medium heat setting.
- As the mixture thickens, stir in the sweetener (about .5 tbsp.).
- Serve with your favorite garnishes but count those carbs.

## Porridge with Cinnamon and Hemp Hearts

**Serving Yields**: 1

**Nutritional Counts**: Net Carbs: 3.6 g| Fat: 13.3 g

**Ingredients:**

- Freshly ground flaxseeds – 2 tbsp.
- Almond milk – unsweetened – 1 cup
- Alcohol-free stevia – 5 drops
- Chia seeds – 1 tbsp.
- Pure vanilla extract - .75 tsp.
- Hemp hearts - .5 cup
- Ground cinnamon - .5 tsp.

**Ingredients for the toppings:**

- Hemp hearts – 1 tbsp.
- Crushed almonds - .25 cup
- Brazil nuts - 3

**Preparation Method:**

- Combine the fixings (omit the toppings for now) using a saucepan over medium heat.
- Once the toppings are gently boiling; stir and continue cooking for another 2 minutes.
- Take the pan from the burner and add the almonds and garnish with the hemp hearts and Brazil nuts.
- Enjoy this yummy delight and prepare for your day!

# Chapter 2: Delicious Meals and Salads

## Meals

### Asparagus and Mushrooms with Cauliflower Risotto

**Serving Yields**: 2

**Nutritional Counts**: Net Carbs: 9 g| Fat: 14 g

**Ingredients:**

- Large onion - .5 of 1
- Cauliflower rice – 7.5 oz.
- Garlic clove - 1
- Olive oil – 2 tbsp.
- Asparagus – 3 oz.
- Mushrooms – 4 oz.

- Lemon juice – 1 tbsp.
- White wine – 3 tbsp.
- Lemon zest - .5 of 1
- Parsley – finely chopped – 2 tbsp.

**Preparation Method:**

- Prep the veggies by mincing the garlic and dicing the onions. Trim the asparagus into ½-inch pieces and slice the mushrooms.
- Saute the garlic and onions in a hot skillet with the oil for 3-5 minutes. Toss in the mushrooms and continue cooking slowly for another minute.
- Blend in the asparagus and cook for 2-3 minutes. Pour in the wine, lemon juice, and cauliflower rice.
- Cook until tender for approximately 5-10 minutes.
- Season to your liking and serve.

## Asparagus and Tofu Stir Fry

**Serving Yields:** 3

**Nutritional Counts:** Net Carbs: 22 g| Fat: 24 g

**Ingredients:**

- Sliced extra-firm tofu – 8 oz.
- Ginger – peeled and grated – 1 tbsp.
- Sesame oil – 1-2 spritz
- Thinly sliced green onions - 4

- Toasted and chopped cashew nuts – 1 handful
- Tripped and chopped asparagus – 1 bunch
- Hoisin sauce – 2 tbsp.
- Basil -1 handful
- Mint - 1 handful
- Zest and juice – 1 lime
- Chopped spinach – 3 handfuls
- Salt – 1 pinch
- Chopped garlic cloves - 3

**Preparation Method:**

- Prepare a wok with the oil and cook the tofu a few minutes. Place on a platter.
- Warm more oil and sauté the pepper flakes, with the asparagus, onions, salt, and grated ginger. Cook 1 minute.
- Toss in the cashews, garlic, and spinach. Continue cooking 1-2 minutes.
- Add the tofu back in the mixture and add the lime juice, zest, and hoisin sauce.
- Continue stir-frying for another 20 seconds.
- Arrange on a serving platter and garnish with the mint and basil.

## Broccoli Noodles and Tofu

**Serving Yields**: 3

**Nutritional Counts**: Net Carbs: 14 g| Fat: 18 g

**Ingredients:**

- Broccoli stems – 2 spiralized
- EVOO – 2 tbsp.
- Diced onion - .5 of 1
- Extra-firm tofu - 1 block - 14 oz.
- Minced cloves of garlic - 2
- Finely diced red bell pepper - 1
- Cumin – 1 tsp.
- Turmeric – 1 tsp.
- Pepper and Salt – to taste

**Preparation Method:**

- After a pot of water starts boiling, add the broccoli. Cook until done or about 2-3 minutes.

- Warm up a pan with the oil. Once it is hot, start sautéing the onions, peppers, and garlic for three to four minutes. Stir in the cumin and cook 1 minute.

- Lastly, stir in the rest of the fixings and cook two to three minutes.

- Divide into three servings and enjoy.

## Cauliflower Tabbouleh

**Serving Yields**: 8

**Nutritional Counts**: Net Carbs: 5.3 g| Fat: 7.19 g

**Ingredients:**

- Lightly steamed cauliflower rice – 2 cups

- Fresh mint – 1 cup

- Fresh parsley – 1 cup

- English cucumber - 1

- Red bell pepper - 1

- Cherry tomatoes - .5 lb.

- Red onion - 1

- EVOO - .25 cup

- Pepper and salt to taste

- Lemon juice - .25 cup

**Preparation Method:**

- This is such a healthy treat. All it takes is adding the fixings into a bowl to toss.
- Serve and enjoy anytime.

## Collard Green Wraps

**Serving Yields**: 1

**Nutritional Counts**: Net Carbs: 3.1 g| Fat: 8.4 g

Ingredients:

- Sliced carrots - .25 cup
- Deveined collard greens - 2
- Sauerkraut -2 tbsp.
- Tahini sauce - 2 tbsp.

**Preparation Method:**

- Combine the sauerkraut and carrots and place inside the collard leaves.
- Roll it into a wrap and drizzle with the sauce.

## Crispy Tofu and Cauliflower Rice

**Serving Yields**: 2

**Nutritional Counts**: Net Carbs: 31.5 g| Fat: 34 g

**Ingredients for the Stir-Fry:**

- Toasted sesame oil – 1 tbsp.
- Extra-firm tofu - organic – 12 oz.
- Garlic cloves - 2 or 1 tbsp. minced
- Head cauliflower – 1 Small

**Ingredients for the Sauce:**

- Low-sodium soy sauce or tamari - .25 cup
- Toasted sesame oil- 1.5 tbsp.
- Light brown sugar – or another substitute - .25 cup
- <u>C</u><u>hili garlic sauce</u> - .5 tsp.
- Natural almond butter - salted – 2.5 tbsp.

**Optional Ingredients**

- Veggies: Green onion, baby Bok choy, broccoli, red pepper, etc.
- *Suggested Toppings:* Cilantro, freshly squeezed lime juice, or sriracha

**Preparation Method:**

- Drain the tofu about 1 1/2 hours before you plan to have dinner. Trim the bok down if it's larger than 12 ounces.
- Roll the tofu in an absorbent towel several times. Put a heavy object on top to press it down. Place something like a cutting board with heavy canned goods or similar objects; anything to add more weight. Do this for about 15 minutes.
- Warm up the oven to 400°F and cube the tofu. Prepare a baking tin with a single sheet of parchment paper. Bake for 25 minutes until it has firmed up. When done, set it aside to cool.

- Whisk the sauce fixings together until well mixed. Adjust the seasonings to your liking. Try adding a little more peanut butter to taste. Marinate to saturate the tofu or about 15 minutes.
- Meanwhile, rice the cauliflower using a food processor or large grater. Set it aside.

- Smash the garlic and prep the vegetables. Use the medium-high temperature setting and add the veggies. Cook them now in a dash of soy sauce and sesame oil. When done, cover them to keep warm.
- Spoon the tofu into the preheated pan with several spoonfuls of the sauce to cover. Continue cooking until browned. When done, set aside.
- Prepare the same skillet and spritz with some of the sesame oil. Toss in the riced cauliflower and garlic. Cover and steam the rice for about five to eight minutes or until tender and lightly browned and tender. Add more sauce and stir well.
- Serve the rice topped with tofu and the prepared vegetables.

## Eggplant Lasagna

**Serving Yields**: 4

**Nutritional Counts**: Net Carbs: 4 g| Fat: 8 g

**Ingredients:**

- Sliced eggplant – 1
- Marinara sauce – 1 cup
- Salt – 1 tbsp.
- Vegan cheese of choice - .5 cup
- Vegan cashew ricotta – 1 cup
- Olive oil – as needed

**Preparation Method:**

- Shake the salt over the eggplant rounds and set to the side for an hour. Rinse and pat them dry.
- Lightly spritz a baking dish with the oil and layer the sliced eggplant on the bottom. Brush with the sauce and sprinkle with the cheese.
- Add another layer of eggplant, ricotta, and lastly the marinara sauce. Make one more layer of the eggplant, sauce, and cheese.
- Bake with a lid on for 1/2 hour. Take the cover off and continue cooking for another 15 minutes before serving.

## Falafel with Tahini Sauce

**Serving Yields:** 2

**Nutritional Counts:** Net Carbs: 5 g| Fat: 24 g

**Ingredients:**

- Raw pureed cauliflower – 1 cup or 1 med head - florets only

- Ground coriander - .5 tbsp.
- Ground cumin – 1 tbsp.
- Ground slivered almonds - .5 cup
- Kosher salt – 1 tsp.
- Minced garlic clove - 1
- Cayenne pepper - .5 tsp.
- Large eggs - 2
- Freshly chopped parsley – 2 tbsp.
- Coconut flour – 3 tbsp.

**Ingredients for the Tahini Sauce:**

- Water – 4 tbsp.
- Tahini paste – 2 tbsp.
- Salt – 1 tsp.
- Minced garlic clove -
- Lemon juice – 1 tbsp.
- For Cooking: Olive or grapeseed oil

**Preparation Method:**

- Use a food processor and puree enough cauliflower to make one cup with a grainy texture. Process the almonds the same way, but don't over grind. Combine the fixings in a mixing bowl and add the remainder of the components of the recipe until well blended.

- Warm up a half mixture of olive and grape seed oil. Make (eight) three-inch patties and add to the pan.

- Cook until browned and turn them over. Four minutes for each side should be sufficient. Add them to a platter to drain on some paper towels.

- Mix all of the tahini fixings in a bowl, adding small portions of water a little at a time until it reaches the desired thickness.

- Use the tahini sauce as a garnish with the tomato and parsley.

## French Style Ratatouille

**Serving Yields**: 10

**Nutritional Counts**: Net Carbs: 9 g| Fat: 25 g

**Ingredients:**

- Eggplants – 2
- Tomatoes - 4
- Thyme sprigs - 4
- Zucchinis - 8
- Olive oil – 2 tbsp.
- Basil - .25 cup
- Garlic cloves - 3
- Yellow onions - 2
- Bell peppers - 3
- Salt – to your liking
- Bay leaf - 1

**Preparation Method:**

- Prepare the veggies. Peel and cube the eggplant. Dice the onions and mince the cloves. Chop the rest of the vegetables.
- Toss the eggplant with salt in a colander. Let it rest a few minutes.
- Warm up a Dutch oven with 1 teaspoon of oil. Sauté the onions for 10 minutes and add the salt. Add to the eggplant bowl. Rinse and squeeze all the water from the eggplant and cook 10 minutes in the Dutch oven. Add to the veggie dish.
- Warm up the rest of the oil and sauté the garlic. Add the tomatoes, thyme sprigs, and bay leaves.
- Be sure to deglaze the bottom. Toss in the veggies and mix well.
- Simmer and lower the heat setting for 45 minutes. Stir occasionally.
- Trash the bay leaf and thyme when done and stir in the basil.
- Serve for a very healthy meal for lunch or dinner.

# Green Panini

**Serving Yields**: 1

**Nutritional Counts**: Net Carbs: 35.51 g| Fat: 55.21 g

**Ingredients:**

- Baby spinach – 1 cup
- Low-carb bread – 2 slices
- Pesto – 4 tbsp.
- Sliced avocado - .5 of 1
- Vegan butter – 1 tbsp.
- Pepper and salt – to your liking
- Hot sauce – 1-2 spritz

**Preparation Method:**

- Use a knife to spread butter onto each slice of bread (only on one side). Spread pesto on the other side.
- Add one slice in a skillet (low heat). Add some salt and pepper. Top it off with the avocado and spinach.
- Add the slice of bread with the butter side facing out. Prepare until golden brown (3-4 min.). Flip and do the same.
- Drizzle with the hot sauce and enjoy right away!

# Sesame Tofu and Eggplant

**Serving Yields**: 4

**Nutritional Counts**: Net Carbs: 6.87 g| Fat: 24.45 g

## Ingredients:

- Firm tofu block – 1 lb.
- Fresh cilantro - chopped – 1 cup
- Toasted sesame oil – 4 tbsp.
- Minced red pepper flakes – 1 tsp.
- Finely minced garlic– 2 cloves
- <u>Swerve confectioners</u> – 2 tsp.
- Eggplant -1 whole
- Unseasoned rice vinegar – 3 tbsp.
- Olive oil – 1 tbsp.
- To Taste – Salt and pepper
- Sesame seeds - .25 cup
- Soy sauce - .25 cup

## Preparation Method:

- Warm up the oven to 200°F. take the tofu block from the package and wrap it with a few paper towels

- Place a heavy object such as a platter or cutting board with books or similar items on top. Let the water be pressed out.

- Place the minced garlic, 2 tablespoons of the sesame oil, the cilantro, pepper flakes, the rice vinegar, and sweetener into a large mixing bowl. Combine each of the components well.

- Discard the peel from the eggplant. Julienne the eggplant with a mandolin with a julienne attachment – for a uniform-looking noodle. Toss the marinade and eggplant together.

- Pour the oil into a frying pan using the med-low temperature setting. Let the eggplant simmer until softened. You might need to add a little bit more oil, but remember to adjust the carbs or fats.

- Turn off the oven and mix in the rest of the cilantro with the eggplant. Fold in the noodles to an oven-safe baking dish. Cover with a lid or a sheet of aluminum foil. Set it in the oven to keep warm.

- Warm up the frying pan and slice the tofu into eight slices. Dip the tofu into some of the sesame seeds. Add two tbsp. of the sesame oil into the skillet. Fry both sides of the tofu for 5 seconds until they're crunchy.

- Pour about 1/4 cup of soy sauce into the pan. Cover the pieces of tofu. Cook until the slices until they appear browned and caramelized with the soy sauce.

- Remove the noodles from the oven and plate the tofu on top.

# Salads

## Arugula and Blueberry Salad

**Serving Yields**: 6

**Nutritional Counts**: Net Carbs: 8 g| Fat: 10 g

**Ingredients:**

- Blueberries – 2 cups
- Arugula – 10 oz.
- Dijon mustard – 1 tbsp.
- Avocado oil - .25 cup
- Freshly squeezed orange juice – 2 tbsp.
- Balsamic vinegar – 2 tbsp.

**Preparation Method:**

- Toss the arugula and berries into a salad dish.
- Whisk the rest of the fixings in another cup.
- Toss the dressing and salad together when it's time to eat.

## Asian Zucchini Salad

**Serving Yields**: 10

**Nutritional Counts**: Net Carbs: 3.6 g| Fat: 9.3 g

### Ingredients:
- Shredded cabbage – 1 lb.
- Thinly spiralized zucchini – 1
- Shelled sunflower seeds – 1 cup
- Sliced almonds – 1 cup
- Stevia drops – 1 tsp.
- Avocado oil - .75 cup
- White vinegar - .33 cup

### Preparation Method:
- Toss the cabbage, zucchini, sunflower seeds, and almonds in a salad dish.
- Whisk the stevia, oil, and vinegar.
- Toss the salad and drizzle with the delicious dressing.
- Place in the refrigerator to get cold for about two hours before dinnertime.

# Asparagus and Artichoke Salad

**Serving Yields**: 4

**Nutritional Counts**: Net Carbs: 7.93 g| Fat: 28.06 g

**Ingredients:**

- Artichoke hearts in oil – drain and wedge – 8
- Asparagus – 1 bunch
- Green beans - .5 lb.
- Capers – 1 tbsp.
- Freshly chopped oregano – 2 tsp.
- Toasted pine nuts - .25 cup
- Minced cloves of garlic – 2
- Olive oil - .25 cup
- Pepper and salt – as desired
- Lemon juice – 2 tbsp.

**Preparation Method:**

- Chop the asparagus and green beans into strips. Drain and chop the capers and artichoke hearts.
- Add a pinch of salt to a soup pot of water. Add the green beans and asparagus into the boiling water for 45 seconds. Drain in a mesh colander.
- Add to a pot for an ice-water bath. Once they are chilled, just pat them dry with paper towels.
- Toss all of the fixings into dishes and serve.

# Avocado and Greens Salad

**Serving Yields**: 4

**Nutritional Counts**: Net Carbs: 7.8 g| Fat: 13.9 g

**Ingredients:**

- Mixed baby greens – 4 cups
- Sliced red onion – 1 tbsp.
- Sliced tomato – 1
- Peeled and sliced Haas avocado – 1
- Sliced cucumber – 1

**Dressing Ingredients:**

- Naval orange - .5 of 1
- Lime – 1
- Extra-virgin olive oil – 2 tbsp.
- A crushed clove of garlic – 1
- Oregano – 1 pinch
- To Taste: Freshly cracked pepper and salt

**Preparation Method:**

- Toss all of the salad fixings into a salad dish or individuals bowls for a more accurate measurement.
- Whisk the dressing ingredients well in another container.
- When you are ready to eat, add the dressing, and enjoy!

## Avocado Papaya Salad

**Serving Yields**: 6

**Nutritional Counts**: Net Carbs: 4.4 g| Fat: 8.4 g

### Ingredients:

- Lime juice – 2 tbsp.
- Red onion – chopped – 2 tbsp.
- Diced Haas avocado – 2
- Chopped cilantro – 2 tbsp.
- To Taste – Pepper and Salt

### Preparation Method:

- Combine each of the fixings into individual dishes or one large one.
- Serve when you're ready and enjoy.

## Bell Pepper and Asparagus Salad

**Serving Yields**: 6

**Nutritional Counts**: Net Carbs: 5.1 g| Fat: 23.4 g

### Ingredients:

- Sliced red onion – 1
- Sweet mini peppers – 17.5 oz.

- Freshly chopped asparagus – 14 oz.
- Apple cider vinegar – 3 tbsp.
- Extra-virgin olive oil - .5 cup
- Dijon mustard – 1 tbsp.
- Lemon – 1 zested
- Chopped bell pepper – 1 tsp.
- Finely chopped capers – 2 tbsp.
- Rosemary – 1 tbsp.
- Thyme – 1 tbsp.
- Himalayan salt – 1 tsp.
- Chopped walnuts - .5 cup

**Preparation Method:**

- Thinly slice the mini peppers and dice the asparagus into small chunks. Slice the onion and finely chop the capers, rosemary, and thyme.
- Combine all of the vegetables into a rimmed baking tin.
- Whisk the rest of the fixings until thoroughly combined. Pour about 3/4 of the dressing into the veggies and toss.
- Roast in the hot oven for 15 minutes.
- Stir once or twice and broil for 5 to 6 minutes.

## Caesar Vegan Salad

**Serving Yields:** 4

**Nutritional Counts:** Net Carbs: 5.2 g| Fat: 12.5 g

### Ingredients:

- Ripe avocado - 1
- Lemon juice – 3 tbsp.
- Water – 2 tbsp.
- Garlic cloves - minced – 3
- Capers – 1 tbsp.
- Caper brine – 1 tbsp.
- Dijon mustard – 2 tsp.
- Hemp seeds - .25 cup
- Sea salt and fresh ground pepper, to taste
- Chopped romaine leaves – 12 cups

### Preparation Method:

- Add the lemon juice, avocado, water, garlic, capers, brine, mustard, salt and pepper to the blender or food processor. Blend until smooth.
- You can add a little water if it's too thick. It will look similar to the consistency of pudding. Keep it this way to maintain the ultra-creaminess.
- Spoon the dressing into a container and mix in the hemp seeds for that touch of parmesan similarity.
- Arrange some of the lettuce in a large salad bowl. Spritz with the dressing and rotate the leaves to cover fully.
- Serve immediately.

## Courgette Salad and Herbed Vinaigrette

**Serving Yields**: 4

**Nutritional Counts**: Net Carbs: 1 g| Fat: 6 g

### Ingredients:

- Olive oil – 2 tbsp.

- Lemon juiced – 1
- Chives- chopped - .5 of 1 pkg.
- Chopped mint - .5 of 1 pkg.
- Spiralized courgettes – 10.5 oz.
- To Your Liking: Pepper and salt

**Preparation Method:**

- Use a spiralizer for the courgettes/zucchini.
- Mix the oil with the pepper, salt, and lemon juice. Stir in the herbs.
- Toss the noodles and dressing into a salad dish.
- Toss and serve.

## Eggplant Salad

**Serving Yields**: 6

**Nutritional Counts**: Net Carbs: 6 g| Fat: 9.4 g

**Ingredients:**

- Mashed cloves of garlic – 4
- Eggplants – 4
- Lemon juiced – 1
- Juiced white onion – 1
- Olive oil - .25 cup
- Chopped parsley – 1 handful
- Salt - .5 tsp.

**Preparation Method:**

- Warm up the oven to reach 350°F.
- Roast the eggplants for 45 minutes to one hour.
- Whisk the parsley, garlic, olive oil, onion juice, and lemon juice. Together.
- Scoop the flesh from the eggplants when done.
- Combine the oil mixture with the salt. Stir well.

## Kale Salad and Blueberry Dressing

**Serving Yields:** 6

**Nutritional Counts:** Net Carbs: 10.5 g| Fat: 16 g

## Ingredients:

- Freshly squeezed lime juice – 1 tbsp.
- Curly kale leaves – 6 cups – roughly torn
- Olive oil – 1 tsp.
- Ground black pepper - .5 tsp.
- Sea salt - .5 tsp.
- Avocado – 1
- Apple – 1
- Fresh blueberries - .25 cup
- Shelled and toasted pumpkin seeds – unsalted – 3 tbsp.
- Feta cheese from goat's milk - .25 cup - optional

## Dressing Ingredients:

- Olive oil – 3 tbsp.
- Fresh blueberries - .25 cup
- Freshly minced ginger – 1 tsp.
- Raw honey – 1 tsp.
- Apple cider vinegar – 2 tbsp.
- Freshly cracked black pepper - .25 tsp.
- Sea salt - .25 tsp.
- Water – 3 tbsp.

## Preparation Method:

- Peel the apple and avocado. Remove the pit from the avocado. Dice both.

- Combine the dressing fixings in a blender until creamy.
- Combine the kale with the lime juice, pepper, salt, and oil. Use your hands and massage until wilted.
- Arrange the kale on a serving dish and toss in the rest of the goodies.
- Spritz with the salad dressing.

## Lemony Brussel Sprout Salad

**Serving Yields**: 4

**Nutritional Counts**: Net Carbs: 2.5 g| Fat: 7 g

**Ingredients:**

- Brussel sprouts - 6 oz.
- Lemon – 1 – juiced
- Olive oil – 2 tbsp.
- Freshly ground black pepper and Kosher salt – as desired

**Preparation Method:**

- Rinse the sprouts and trim away the ends. Slice them into halves and dice into fine bits.
- Add to sprouts to a salad platter and toss with the rest of the fixings.
- Serve, smile, and enjoy.

## Pear and Dates with Special Cider Dressing

**Serving Yields**: 4

**Nutritional Counts**: Net Carbs: 11.5 g| Fat: 25.6 g

### Ingredients:

- Sliced fresh pear - .5 of 1
- Romaine lettuce – 2 cups
- Chopped and pitted Medjool dates – 2
- Walnuts – 1 handful
- Topping: Omega croutons

### Dressing Ingredients:

- Olive oil - .25 cup
- Avocado – 1
- Ginger – 1 tbsp.
- Pitted Medjool dates - 2
- Water – 3 tbsp.
- Lemon juice – 2 tbsp.
- Dijon mustard- 1 tbsp.
- Herbamare - .25 tsp.

### Preparation Method:

- Combine all of the dressing fixings in the blender and combine until smooth.
- Toss the salad components into salad dishes and add the dressing.
- Add the croutons if using and serve.

## Pecan Cauliflower Salad

**Serving Yields**: 8

**Nutritional Counts**: Net Carbs: 5.5 g| Fat: 9.2 g

**Ingredients:**

- Red and Yellow pepper - .5 cup of each
- Sliced thin purple cauliflower – 1
- Curly fresh kale – 4 cups – stem removed
- Chopped scallions - .5 cup
- Lemon juice – 1 cup
- Toasted – chopped pecans - .5 cup
- Olive oil – 3 tbsp.
- Pepper and salt to your liking

**Preparation Method:**

- Chop the veggies and remove the stem from the kale.
- Toss all of the fixings into a salad dish and serve.

## Simple Green Salad with Lemon Vinaigrette

**Serving Yields**: 1

**Ingredients for the dressing:**

- Good quality olive oil or extra virgin oil - .25 cup

- Lemon juice – 3-4 cups
- Maple syrup – 1 tsp.
- Salt and black pepper – 1 pinch
- Optional: Minced shallot – 3 tbsp.

**Ingredients for the salad**:
- Organic mixed greens - 5 oz.
- Baby tomatoes - .25 cup
- Thinly sliced shallot or red onion - .25 cup
- Shredded carrots - .5 cup
- Optional: Pomegranate arils or dried fruit - .25 cup
- Salt and pepper - 1 pinch of each
- Toasted pepitas or sunflower seeds - 2 tbsp.

**Preparation Method:**
- First, prepare the dressing by adding all of the fixings to a mixing bowl or into a small blender. Whisk or blend to thoroughly combine.
- Taste and adjust the seasonings as needed by adding more maple syrup for sweetness, lemon for acidity, or salt or pepper to taste. Set aside.
- Prepare the salad by adding the rinsed greens to a serving bowl or platter and topping with baby tomatoes, shallot or onion, carrots, pomegranate arils or dried fruit (optional), a pinch of salt and pepper, and toasted pepitas or sunflower seeds.
- Add the dressing to the salad and toss to coat, or serve on the side. It's best when fresh.
- Store salad separate from dressing if keeping for later use. Will keep in the refrigerator up to 2-3 days. Store the dressing in the refrigerator 3-4 days. The oil can harden when cold, so let set out for a few minutes to warm and shake well to incorporate before serving leftovers.

## Sun-Dried Tomato Salad and Cider Dressing

**Serving Yields**: 2

**Nutritional Counts**: Net Carbs: 11.3 g| Fat: 16.2 g

## Ingredients:

- Chopped cucumber - .5 of 1
- Sun-dried tomatoes in the oil – 2 tbsp.
- Shaved carrots - 3
- Thinly sliced red pepper – 1
- Sunflower seeds – 1 tsp.

## Dressing Ingredients:

- Dijon mustard – 1 tsp.
- Sunflower oil – 1 tsp.
- Apple cider vinegar – 1 tsp.
- Dried oregano - .25 tsp.
- Dried basil - .25 tsp.
- White powdered stevia – 1 pinch
- Herbamare - .125 tsp.

## Preparation Method:

- Toss all of the veggies into a salad mixing dish along with the sunflower seeds.
- Whisk the dressing fixings well.
- Pour the dressing over the tossed salad and serve.

## Thai Peanut Zucchini Noodle Salad

**Serving Yields**: 4

**Nutritional Counts:** Net Carbs: 8 g| Fat: 12 g

## Ingredients:

- Medium zucchini - 3 spiralized
- Carrot – 1 spiralized
- Chopped green onions - .25 cup
- Extra firm tofu, drained and cubed - .5 of 1 block
- Skinny Peanut Sauce - .5 cup (+) 1-2 tbsp. water
- Peanuts - .5 cup

## for the SKINNY SAUCE:

**Serving Yields:** 18

**Nutritional Counts:** Net Carbs: 8 g| Fat: 12 g

## Ingredients for the sauce:

- Protein Plus HYPERLINK "https://www.amazon.com/gp/product/B0052OOYOW/ref=as_li_tl?ie=UTF8&camp=1789&creative=9325&creativeASIN=B0052OOYOW&linkCode=as2&tag=vega05-20&linkId=8671ed905d4daf99a65cd5d7131e6cf3"peanut flour - .25 cup
- Ginger – 1 tsp.
- Garlic powder - .5 tsp.
- Low-sodium soy sauce - gluten-free, if desired – 2 tbsp.
- Lakanto Liquid Monkfruit Sweetener or another liquid sweetener - 6 drops or to taste

- Lime juice - juice of 2 limes - 1 tbsp.
- Water - add more if desired – 2 tbsp.

**Ingredients for the salad:**

- Spiralized carrot- <u>1</u>
- Medium spiralized zucchini - 3
- Diced green onions - .25 cup
- Extra-firm tofu - .5 of a block
- <u>Skinny Peanut Sauce</u>- .5 cup plus 1-2 Tbsp water
- Peanuts - .5 cup

**Preparation Method:**

- Drain and cube the tofu. Prepare <u>the sauce</u> by adding the water until it's like you like it.
- Combine the remainder of the fixings except for the peanuts in another container.
- Top it off with the prepared salad dressing, and toss well. Sprinkle using some of the peanuts, and serve.

# Chapter 3: Healthy Soups – Stews and Chowder

## Beetroot Ginger Soup

**Serving Yields**: 2

**Nutritional Counts**: Net Carbs: 5 g| Fat: 12 g

**Ingredients:**

- 
- Coconut milk - .5 of 1 can
- Chopped beetroots - 4
- Chopped onion – 1 peeled
- Fresh ginger - peeled and chopped – 3 tbsp.

- Black pepper and salt - .5 tsp. of ea.
- Coconut oil – 1 tbsp.
- Vegetable stock – 3 cups
- Garlic cloves - 3 minced

**Preparation Method:**

- Warm up a saucepan and add the oil. Slowly cook the onion 3-4 minutes.
- Toss in the garlic and ginger. Sauté another 2 minutes.
- Whisk the vegetable stock and beetroot together. Once it begins to simmer, just lower the heat. Simmer for about 20 minutes with a lid on the pot.
- When done, remove from the burner and add the milk, pepper, and salt.
- Make it creamy smooth with an immersion blender.

## Broccoli and Cauliflower Soup

**Serving Yields**: 2

**Nutritional Counts**: Net Carbs: 6.1 g| Fat: 7.7 g

**Ingredients:**

- Cauliflower – 3.5 oz.
- Broccoli – 3.5 oz.
- Olive oil – 2 tsp.
- Chopped onion – 1 oz.
- Coconut milk - .25 cup
- White pepper and Pink salt – to your liking

**Preparation Method:**

- Finely chop the broccoli and cauliflower.

- Warm up a pan with the oil. Slowly add the onions and cook slowly until they are fragrant and translucent. Toss in the cauliflower, pepper, salt, and diluted coconut milk.

- Pour in 1/2 of the broccoli and simmer 5-7 additional minutes. Let it cool a minute or so, and puree with an immersion blender.

- Fold in the remainder of the broccoli.

- Serve and enjoy!

## Cabbage and Beet Soup

**Serving Yields**: 4

**Nutritional Counts**: Net Carbs: 6 g| Fat: 7 g

**Ingredients:**

- 
- Shredded green cabbage – 2 cups
- Beets – 1 cup
- Carrots – 1 cup
- Olive oil – 2 tbsp.
- Vegetable stock – 3 cups
- Lemon juice – 1 tbsp.
- Garlic powder - .5 tsp.
- Onion powder - .5 tsp.

- Bay leaves - 2
- Juniper berries – 1 tbsp.
- Pepper and salt – to your liking

**Preparation Method:**

- Shred the cabbage, beets, and carrots.
- Warm up a saucepan with the oil. When it's hot, toss in the cabbage, carrots, and beets. Sauté 5 minutes.
- Blend in the rest of the fixings and continue cooking until tender.
- Strain out the juniper berries and bay leaves.
- Let cool before serving.

## Chili – Vegan Style

**Serving Yields**: 4

**Nutritional Counts**: Net Carbs: 2 g| Fat: 14 g

**Ingredients:**

- 
- Green bell pepper - 1
- Red bell pepper – 1
- Textured vegetable protein – 2.5 oz.
- Soy sauce – keto-friendly – 1 tbsp.
- Vegetable oil – 1 tbsp.
- Diced canned tomatoes – 14 oz.

- Cooked black soybeans – 2 cups
- Minced cloves of garlic – 5
- Veggie broth - .5 cup
- Smoked paprika powder - .5 tsp.
- Oregano - .5 tsp.
- Chili powder - .5 tsp.

**Preparation Method:**

- Dice the peppers and set aside.
- Toss the vegetable protein into the saucepan and submerge it with water.
- Warm up the oil in a pot. Sauté the peppers and textured vegetable protein for about five minutes. Whisk in the garlic and sauté one minute. Stir in the rest of the fixings.
- Once boiling, lower the heat and simmer for 10-15 minutes.
- Serve.

## Chilled Minty Avocado Soup

**Serving Yields**: 2

**Nutritional Counts**: Net Carbs: 4 g| Fat: 26 g

**Ingredients:**

- Romaine lettuce leaves - 2
- Ripe avocado - 1

- Lime juice – 1 tbsp.
- Chilled coconut milk – 1 cup
- Salt – to your liking
- Fresh mint leaves - 20

**Preparation Method:**
- Add all of the fixings to a blender.
- Mix well until creamy smooth.
- Set aside for about ten minutes to cool.

## Creamy Avocado Soup

**Serving Yields**: 4

**Nutritional Counts**: Net Carbs: 7 g| Fat: 31 g

**Ingredients:**
- Broccoli – florets – 1 head
- Minced garlic cloves - 2
- Chopped onion – 1
- Coconut oil – 2 tbsp.
- Vegetable stock – 1 cup
- Bay leaf - 1
- Coconut milk – 2 cups
- Pepper and salt – to your liking

**Preparation Method:**

- Warm up a saucepan with the oil. When it's hot, add the onion and garlic. Sauté 5-6 minutes. Toss in the rest of the fixings.

- Once it starts to boil; lower the heat setting and simmer approximately 15-20 minutes. Trash the bay leaf.

- Blend with an immersion blender and serve.

## Creamy Red Gazpacho Soup

**Serving Yields**: 6

**Nutritional Counts**: Net Carbs: 8.5 g| Fat: 50.8 g

**Ingredients:**

- 
- Medium tomatoes – 4-5
- Red peppers – 1 large
- Small green peppers – 2
- Medium avocados - 2
- Small red onion - 1
- Cloves of garlic - 2
- Fresh lemon juice - 2 tbsp.
- Wine vinegar/apple cider - 2 tbsp.
- Freshly chopped parsley - 2-4 tbsp.
- Medium spring onions – 2
- Freshly chopped basil - 2-4 tbsp.
- Large cucumber - 1

- Salt – such as Himalayan rock salt – 1 tsp.
- To your liking: Freshly cracked black pepper
- Feta cheese– 7.1 oz.
- EVOO – 1 cup
- Also needed: Parchment paper

**Preparation Method:**

- Program the oven to 400°F.
- Slice the peppers in half and deseed. Arrange them cut side down on parchment paper and roast them for approximately 20 minutes. The skin will turn black and blister.
- Meanwhile, chop the red onion and add to a pot. Cut up the tomatoes into quarter sections, and cut the avocado in half and deseed; adding each to the pot with the onions.
- Take the peppers out of the oven and cool. Throw away the skins and toss into the pot. Blend in the garlic, fresh herbs, olive oil, pepper, salt, vinegar, and lemon juice. Pulse with a hand mixer until smooth. (Reserve a bit of the oil for garnishing.)
- Dice the onion and cucumber, and add to the soup mixing well, seasoning to taste as desired.
- Serve and top with some fresh herbs, and a drizzle of olive oil (about 1 tablespoon for each serving).
- *Note*: You can mix and match the types of peppers to change the coloring of the soup.

## Creamy Tomato Soup

**Serving Yields**: 4

**Nutritional Counts**: Net Carbs: 7.7 g| Fat: 15.9 g

**Ingredients:**

- Sun-dried tomatoes - .5 cup
- Raw macadamia nuts - .5 cup
- Roma tomatoes - 4
- White pepper - .5 tsp.
- Sea salt – 1 tsp.
- Black pepper - .25 tsp.
- Garlic clove - 1
- Hot water – 4 cups
- Fresh basil - .25 cup

**Preparation Method:**

- Toss each of the components into a high-speed blender.
- Prepare for 5 minutes.
- Serve in a warm bowl.

## Ginger Cauliflower Stew

**Serving Yields**: 6

**Nutritional Counts:** Net Carbs: 12 g| Fat: 24 g

**Ingredients:**

- Tomatoes – 3
- Onion – 1
- Coconut oil – 2 tbsp.
- Cumin seeds – 1 tsp.
- Chopped kale – 1 cup
- Cauliflower florets – 1 head
- Jalapeno – seeded – 1
- Cumin powder – 1 tbsp.
- Ginger paste – 2 tsp.
- Turmeric powder – 1 tsp.
- Coriander powder – 1 tbsp.
- Coconut milk – full-fat unsweetened – 1 can
- Chopped cilantro – 2 tbsp.
- Sea salt – 1 tsp.

**Preparation Method:**

- Finely chop the kale, jalapeno, tomatoes, and onions. Separate the cauliflower into florets.

- Warm up the oil in a soup pot and toss in the cumin seeds. Sauté the onions 1 minute and fold in the tomatoes. Simmer a minute or two and add the rest of the fixings.

- Cover the pot and simmer for 15 minutes – making sure to stir after each 5-minute segment.

- Serve and enjoy.

## Mushroom Soup

**Serving Yields**: 5

**Nutritional Counts:** Net Carbs: 6 g| Fat: 21 g

**Ingredients:**

- Olive oil – 1 tbsp.
- Diced onion - .5 of 1
- Sliced mushrooms – 20 oz.
- Minced cloves of garlic - 6
- Coconut cream – 1 cup
- Black pepper - .25 tsp.
- Sea salt - .75 tsp.
- Unsweetened almond milk – 1 cup
- Vegetable broth – 2 cups

**Preparation Method:**

- Warm up a big cooking soup pot. Pour in the oil. Toss in the onions and mushroom. Sauté for 10-15 minutes. Fold in the garlic and cook about one additional minute.
- Fold in the remainder of the fixings and simmer until done (approx. 15 min.). Stir often.
- Before serving, use an immersion blender until it's the desired consistency.

Like what you're reading? Want to hear this as an audio book? Click here to get this book for FREE when you join Audible!!

https://adbl.co/2YmbdC8

## Red Onion Soup

**Serving Yields**: 2

**Nutritional Counts**: Net Carbs: 49.46 g| Fat: 51.91 g

**Ingredients:**

- Garlic cloves - 2
- Red onions - 2
- Lemon juice – 1.5 tbsp.
- Vegetable broth – 2.5 cups
- Olive oil – 5 tbsp.
- Walnuts – 4 tbsp.
- Low-carb bread – 2 slices
- Pepper and salt - to taste
- Pesto – 2 tsp.

**Preparation Method**

- Slice the onions into ringlets and add to a saucepan and half of the oil. Toss in the minced garlic. Sauté 5 minutes and add the juice and broth.

- Sprinkle with the salt and pepper and simmer with the lid on the pot for 10 minutes.
- Cube and fry the bread with the walnuts in the remainder of the oil until crispy.
- Top off the hot soup with the walnuts, pesto, and croutons.

## Spanish Soup

**Serving Yields**: 4

**Nutritional Counts**: Net Carbs: 6 g| Fat: 11 g

### Ingredients:

- Tomatoes – 1.5 lb.
- Cucumber - 1
- White onion - .25 of 1
- Green bell pepper - .5 o 1
- Garlic-flavored olive oil – 3 tbsp.
- Black pepper and salt – as desired

### Preparation Method:

- Discard the pepper seeds and chop the cucumber, onion, peppers, and tomatoes. Combine the fixings in a food processor. Mix until smooth.
- Cover and chill in the refrigerator for 1 hour. Serve with a few finely chopped peppers and tomatoes.

## Spinach and Turnip Soup

**Serving Yields**: 2

**Nutritional Counts**: Net Carbs: 4.2 g| Fat: 13.3 g

**Ingredients:**

- Chopped turnips – 1.75 oz.
- Chopped spinach – 5.29 oz.
- Chopped ginger - .25 oz.
- Olive oil – 3 tsp.
- Desiccated coconut – approx. .33 oz.
- Coconut milk - .25 cup
- Water – 2 cups

**Preparation Method:**

- Warm up the oil in a pan on the stovetop and sauté the ginger. Toss in the veggies and let it simmer over the high-temperature setting until the liquids are released.
- Lower the heat and blend in the desiccated coconut.
- Dilute the milk with the water and add to the pan. Simmer on the low heat setting.
- When done, let it cool, and use an immersion blender to cream the soup.
- Enjoy anytime.

## Superfood Keto Soup

**Serving Yields**: 6

**Nutritional Counts**: Net Carbs: 6.8 g| Fat: 37.6 g

**Ingredients:**

- Medium head cauliflower – 1 – 14 oz.
- Medium white onion – 1
- Crumbled bay leaf – 1
- Garlic cloves – 2
- Frozen spinach – 7.8 oz or fresh spinach 7.1 oz. approx.
- Watercress – 5.3 oz.
- Vegetable broth – 1 liter
- Coconut milk – 8 fl. oz.
- Coconut oil - .25 cup
- Pink Himalayan rock salt – 1 tsp.
- Optional fresh herbs such as chives or parsley

**Preparation Method:**

- Remove the skin from the onion and garlic. Dice them into fine bits.
- Toss everything into a Dutch oven or soup pot - lightly greased with coconut oil. Simmer using the med-high heat setting until lightly browned.
- Rinse the watercress and spinach. Sit to the side.
- Dice the cauliflower into small florets and toss into the cooking pot with browned onion and crumbled bay leaf. Simmer for around five minutes.
- Add the spinach and watercress and cook another two to three minutes or until wilted. Pour in the vegetable stock and bring to a boil, cooking until the cauliflower is crisp-tender. Pour in coconut milk adding a shake of pepper and salt. Remove from the burner and pulse with a hand mixer.
- Serve immediately or chill and keep refrigerated for up to five days.
- You can also freeze for longer storage times.

# Thai Pumpkin Soup

**Serving Yields**: 6

**Nutritional Counts**: Net Carbs: 11 g| Fat: 15 g

**Ingredients:**

- Sliced onion - 1
- Grated ginger – 1 tbsp.
- Pumpkin – peeled and chopped – 53 oz. approx.
- Coconut oil – 4 tsp.
- Mashed lemongrass - 1
- Thai red curry paste – 3 tbsp.
- Coconut milk – 1.75 cups
- Vegetable stock – 3.5 cups
- For Seasoning: Lime juice

**Preparation Method:**

- Program the oven setting to 395°F.

- Toss the cubes of pumpkin into 2 teaspoons of the oil and lime juice in a baking pan. Bake 30 minutes.

- Warm up a skillet with the remainder of the oil and sauté the onion, lemongrass, and ginger for 8-10 minutes. Toss in the rest of the fixings and simmer 5 more minutes.

- Remove the lemongrass and cool. Mix well with an immersion blender before serving.

## Turmeric Cabbage Soup

**Serving Yields:** 4

**Nutritional Counts:** Net Carbs: 5 g| Fat: 10 g

**Ingredients:**

- Coconut milk - .25 cup
- White cabbage – 1 head
- Turmeric powder – 2 tsp.
- Coconut oil – 2 tsp.
- Salt and pepper - .5 tsp. of each
- Cumin powder – 1 tsp.
- Vegetable stock – 3 cups
- Garlic cloves - 2

**Preparation Method:**

- Peel and mince the garlic cloves.
- Warm up a skillet and add the oil. Sauté the garlic and cabbage for 10 minutes.
- Empty the stock into the mixture and simmer for 20 minutes (lid on).
- Remove from the burner and stir in the rest of the fixings.
- Prepare with an immersion blender until creamy smooth.
- Tip: Turmeric is known for its health benefits including fighting inflammation and is superb for those who suffer from arthritis.

## Zucchini Basil Soup

**Serving Yields:** 4

**Nutritional Counts**: Net Carbs: 4 g| Fat: 7 g

**Ingredients:**

- Cloves of garlic – 2-3
- Zucchinis - 2
- Onion - 1
- Coconut oil – 2 tbsp.
- Basil leaves - .33 cup
- Pepper and salt - to taste
- Vegetable stock – 3 cups

**Preparation Method:**

- Trim and chop the zucchini, cloves of garlic, and onion.
- Warm the oil in a saucepan. When hot, toss in the onion and garlic. Sauté for 3 min.

- Blend in the zucchini chunks and sauté another 5 min.
- Empty the stock into the mixture and simmer 15 additional minutes.
- At that time, mix in the basil.
- Blend with an immersion blender until creamy.
- Serve and enjoy.

# Chapter 4: Vegan Creams - Sauces and Dips

## Avocado Mayo

**Serving Yields**: 4

**Nutritional Counts**: Net Carbs: 4 g| Fat: 5 g

### Ingredients:

- Avocado - .5 of 1 medium
- Pink salt – 1 pinch
- Ground cayenne pepper - .5 tsp.
- Lime juice - .5 of 1
- Olive oil - .25 cup

### Preparation Method:

- Dice the avocado and toss into a blender or food processor. Pulse and add in the salt, cayenne, cilantro, and lime juice.
- When smooth, stir in the oil – 1 tbsp. at a time - pulsing in between each addition.
- You can store the mayo for up to one week in a sealed glass bottle.

## Barbecue Sauce

**Serving Yields**: 2.5 cups – 2 tbsp. each

### Ingredients:

- Agave nectar or pure maple syrup - 3 tbsp.

- Apple cider vinegar – 2 tbsp.

- Tomato sauce - 1 can – 15-16 oz.

- Molasses or extra syrup – 1 tbsp.

- Tamari - reduced-sodium soy sauce – 2-3 tbsp.

- Basil or dried oregano - 1 tsp.

- Chili powder - 1 tsp.

- Smoked or sweet paprika - 1 tsp.

**Preparation Method:**

- Add all of the ingredients in a large container, whisking thoroughly.
- Let it stand for one hour for all of the tasty flavors to blend fully.

## Coconut Whipped Cream

**Serving Yields**: 8

**Nutritional Counts**: Net Carbs: 2.38 g| Fat: 10.4 g

**Ingredients:**

- Coconut cream – not the milk carton - 1 can
- Powdered sugar – vegan-friendly – 2-4 tsp.

**Preparation Method:**

- Overnight: Refrigerate the cream.

- Scoop the cream from the can – leaving the liquid behind. Use a mixer to beat 1 minute (high setting).

- Add the sugar – to taste- and continue beating for another 4 minutes
- Serve and enjoy chilled.

## Eggplant Bruschetta

**Serving Yields**: 4

**Nutritional Counts**: Net Carbs: 2 g| Fat: 5 g

### Ingredients:

- Eggplant - 1
- Olive oil – 2 tbsp.
- Salt - .5 tsp.
- Pepper – to taste

### Ingredients for the topping:

- Chopped basil – 2 tbsp.
- Diced tomatoes – 2 cups
- Minced garlic cloves - 2
- Olive oil – 1 tbsp.
- Salt and Pepper – to your liking

### Preparation Method:

- Prepare the Veggies: Slice the eggplant in circles. Dice the tomatoes, chop the basil and mince the garlic cloves. Add to a salad bowl.
- Sprinkle with the salt and set aside for ½ hour.
- Grill the eggplant in a preheated grill (4-7 min. per side).

- To serve; brush oil on the grilled eggplant slices and season to your liking.
- Garnish with the topping and enjoy with your gang.

## Guacamole

**Serving Yields**: 4

**Nutritional Counts**: Net Carbs: 5.4 g| Fat: 14.9 g

**Ingredients:**

- Cherry tomatoes – 7 oz.
- Avocados – 2
- White onion - 1
- Red chili pepper - 1
- Garlic cloves - 2
- Lime juice – 2 tbsp.
- Chopped cilantro – 2 tbsp.
- Salt and black pepper - to taste

**Preparation Method:**

- Slice the avocados in half and scoop out the insides.
- Mash and mix it with the rest of the fixings.
- Serve any way you choose.

## Hummus and Avocado

**Serving Yields**: 4

**Nutritional Counts**: Net Carbs: 2.4 g| Fat: 7.2 g

**Ingredients:**

- Lemon – juiced - .5 of 1
- Olive oil – 1 tbsp.
- Zucchini - 1
- Avocado - 1
- Creamy roasted tahini with salt - .25 cup
- Garlic cloves – minced - 3
- Sea salt – 1 tsp.
- Cumin – 1 tsp.

**Preparation Method:**

- Peel and cube the zucchini and avocado. Mince the garlic cloves and add all of the fixings into a food processor. Mix until creamy smooth.
- Let it chill in the fridge for 3-4 hours.
- Serve and enjoy to the side of a veggie platter at your next dinner party!

# Ketchup

**Nutritional Counts**: Net Carbs: 1 g| Fat: -0- g

**Ingredients:**

- Diced tomatoes – 1 can organic – 14.5 oz. (+) 1 can water

- Italian seasoning – 1 tsp.
- Star anise – 1 piece
- White vinegar - .5 tbsp.
- Freshly ground pepper
- Salt
- Optional: Erythritol – to your liking

**Preparation Method:**

- Pour the tomatoes and a can of water into a small pan.
- Stir in the herbs and anise. Simmer using the low heat setting for one hour, stirring frequently.
- Transfer the pan from the heat and add the vinegar. Add any other seasonings as desired and remove the star anise.
- Let it cool and puree into a smooth ketchup sauce using a blender/food processor.
- Tip: Store in the fridge for no more than 4 days.

## Lemon and Jalapeno Cream Sauce

**Serving Yields**: 8

**Nutritional Counts**: Net Carbs: 4.94 g| Fat: 7.08 g

**Ingredients:**

- Raw unsalted cashews - .75 cup
- Lemon juice – 5 tbsp.
- Lemon zest - .5 tsp.

- Fresh jalapeno - 1
- Olive oil - .5 tbsp.
- Cloves of garlic – skins-on - 2
- Unsweetened soy milk - .5 cup
- Salt - .5 tsp.

**Preparation Method:**

- Heat up the oven setting to reach 400°F.
- Soak the cashews for 2-4 hours in water. Line a baking sheet with some parchment paper.
- Slice the jalapenos, remove the seeds, and place on the baking tin with the garlic cloves. Roast for 15 minutes.
- Drain the cashews and add to a blender along with the oil, lemon juice, zest, salt, and soy milk. Toss in the peeled garlic cloves and jalapenos.
- Puree and store in the refrigerator for up to seven days using a closed container.

## Mayo – Vegan Style

**Serving Yields**: 1 cup – 1 tbsp. portions

**Nutritional Counts**: Fat: 13.8 g

**Ingredients:**

- Safflower oil – 1 cup
- Apple cider vinegar – 1 tsp.
- Unsweetened soy milk - .5 cup
- Juiced lemon - 1

- Sea salt - .75 tsp.

**Preparation Method:**

- Use a high-speed blender to mix the lemon juice, soymilk, vinegar, and salt on the high-speed for one minute.
- Slowly pour the oil while blending on low. (Remove the center lid cover.)
- Blend on high with the lid back for about two minutes until thickened.
- Add the mayonnaise to an airtight jar. It needs to chill for a minimum of one hour before using.

## Nutella Spread

**Serving Yields**: 16

**Nutritional Counts**: Net Carbs: 3 g| Fat: 18.7 g

**Ingredients:**

- Roasted almonds - .5 cup
- Roasted hazelnuts – 1 cup
- Macadamia nuts – 1 cup
- Cacao powder -1 tbsp.
- Dark chocolate – 3.5 oz.
- Powdered erythritol – 2 tbsp.
- Virgin coconut oil - 1 tbsp.
- Vanilla powder - .5 tsp.

**Preparation Method:**

- Mix the coconut oil and chocolate in a bowl. Melt using a water bath.
- Use a food processor to turn the nuts into powder. Add the rest of the fixings and process until it reaches the desired texture.

## Peanut Sauce

**Serving Yields**: 6

**Nutritional Counts**: Net Carbs: 6.4 g| Fat: 10.6 g

**Ingredients:**
- Ginger – 1- 5-inch piece
- Garlic cloves - 2
- Tamari - 2 tbsp.
- Water - .25 cup
- Lime juice – 1 tbsp.
- Red pepper flakes - .5 tsp.
- Stevia – 10 drops
- Chopped peanuts - .25 cup
- Chopped green onion – 2 tbsp.
- Natural peanut butter - .5 cup

**Preparation Method**:
- Mix all of the fixings in a blender (omitting the onions and peanuts).
- Mix until creamy and serve with the green onions and peanuts as a topping.

## Portobello Mushroom Bruschetta

**Serving Yields**: 2

**Nutritional Counts**: Net Carbs: 2.48 g| Fat: 37.08 g

**Ingredients:**

- Minced garlic cloves - 6
- Portobello mushrooms - 2
- Olive oil – divided - .33 cup
- Chopped tomatoes - 3
- Chopped basil - .5 cup
- Pepper and Salt – to your liking

**Preparation Method:**

- Combine 2 tbsp. of the oil with 2 garlic cloves in a cup.
- Use a brush of the oil to season the mushrooms. Give the mushrooms a shake of the salt and pepper. Grill for 3 minutes (per side) using medium heat.
- Prepare the basil and tomato mixture with the rest of the olive oil and garlic. Stuff the mushrooms and serve.

## Slow-Cooked Summer Bruschetta

**Serving Yields**: 4

**Nutritional Counts**: Net Carbs: 7.5 g| Fat: 13 g

**Ingredients:**

- Quartered artichoke hearts - .5 cup
- Chopped basil leaves - 6
- Minced garlic – 2 tbsp.
- Capers - .25 cup
- Kalamata olives – halved - .25 cup
- Diced Roma tomatoes - 4
- Avocado oil - 3 tbsp.
- Balsamic vinegar - 3 tbsp.
- Sea salt - .75 tsp.
- Onion powder - .75 tsp.
- Ground black pepper - .5 tsp.

**Preparation Method:**

- Combine all of the fixings in the cooker and mix well.
- Prepare on the high setting for 3 hours. Be sure to stir 2-3 times during the cooking cycle.
- Enjoy this tasty dish alongside your favorite grilled veggies.

## Spinach Avocado Dip

**Serving Yields**: 12

**Nutritional Counts**: Net Carbs: 1.4 g| Fat: 8.8 g

**Ingredients for the dip:**

- Fresh spinach leaves - about 20 large leaves - .5 cup

- Ripened avocado – 2 large or about 2 cups of mashed
- Crushed garlic cloves – 1
- Freshly chopped coriander - .25 cup
- Dairy-free coconut or soy yogurt or another your choice - .75 cup
- Lime juice – 1 tbsp.
- Extra -virgin avocado oil or your favorite – 3 tbsp. (+) more to garnish
- Sea salt - .5 tsp.

**Ingredients for the Mexican Salsa:**
- Cherry tomatoes - a combo of color yellow, red, or orange -10
- Canned red kidney beans - .25 cup
- Chopped fresh coriander – 1 handful to taste
- Ex.-virgin avocado oil – 2 tbsp.
- Lime juice – 1 tbsp.
- Clove of garlic - 1
- Brown Rice Chips – 1 pkg.

**Preparation Method:**

- Trim the fresh spinach leaves. Blanche the leaves by placing them into a large mixing bowl and cover with boiling water. Place a lid on the dish and set aside for two minutes.
- Rinse the spinach using cold water. Squeeze the cooked/blanched spinach leaves to remove all the extra water. Pat them dry on two sheets of absorbent paper towels to remove all the extra water.
- In a food processor, with 'S' blade attachment; add the spinach, mashed ripened avocado, crushed garlic, coriander, coconut yogurt, lime juice, avocado oil, salt, and pepper.
- Process until smooth - about two minutes using the high-speed setting. Transfer into a bowl. Drizzle oil on top if you like.
- Refrigerate at least 30 minutes before serving or before adding the Mexican salsa.
- It stores well in the fridge up to one week in an airtight container. The surface of the dip may change slightly in color - avocado oxidation - simply give a good stir and enjoy.

**Preparation Method for the Salsa:**

- In a mixing bowl, add the red beans and chopped tomatoes.
- Combine with avocado oil, crushed garlic, and lime juice.
- Sprinkle the salsa on top of the dip with extra chopped coriander.
- Serve with a pack of brown rice chips.
- **Tips: Oil Options:** If you don't have avocado oil, any vegetable oil works well, the healthiest alternative will be extra virgin olive oil.

# Tahini and Cilantro Sauce

**Serving Yields**: 4

**Nutritional Counts**: Net Carbs: 4.97 g| Fat: 9.64 g

**Ingredients:**

- Minced garlic cloves - 2
- Tahini - .33 cup
- Water - .25 cup
- Fresh cilantro - .5 cup
- Apple cider vinegar – 1 tbsp.
- Salt - .25 tsp.
- Lemon juice – 1 tsp.

**Preparation Method:**

- Squeeze the lemons for fresh juice.
- Combine all of the components in a blender. Puree and flavor to taste.
- Note: You can refrigerate the sauce for up to two weeks.

# Tofu or Seitan Marinades

**Enjoy the Variety:**

**Serving Yields**: 2 – each marinade is enough for 1 block of tofu or 2 seitan tenders

**Ingredients:**

**BBQ Marinade:**
- BBQ sauce - check to make sure it's vegan – 6 tbsp.
- Liquid smoke - .5 tsp.

**Coconut Curry Marinade:**

- Full-fat coconut milk - .5 cup
- Curry powder – 2 tsp.
- Soy sauce – 2 tbsp.

**Jerk Marinade:**

- Jerk marinade (hot, mild, or a combo) – 3 tbsp.

- Water – 2 tbsp.

## Italian Marinade:

- White wine vinegar or Lemon juice – 2 tbsp.
- Olive oil - 2 tbsp.
- Dried rosemary – 1 tsp.
- Dried basil – 1 tsp.
- Garlic powder - .25 tsp.
- Salt - .25 tsp
- Black pepper - .125 tsp.

## Lemon Mustard Marinade:

- Lemon juice – 2 tbsp.
- Dijon mustard – 2 tbsp.
- Maple syrup or agave – 1 tbsp.
- Black pepper - .125 tsp.

## Sriracha Marinade:

- Sriracha – 2 tbsp.
- Soy sauce or substitute – 1 tbsp.
- Agave or maple syrup - 1 tbsp.

## Sweet Chili Marinade:

- Sweet chili sauce - .25 cup
- Soy sauce – 1 tbsp.

## Balsamic Marinade:

- Olive oil – 2 tbsp.
- Garlic powder - .5 tsp.
- Balsamic vinegar – 2 tbsp.

**Thai Peanut Marinade:**

- Peanut butter – 3 tbsp.
- Lime juice – 1.5 tbsp.
- Soy sauce – 1.5 tbsp.
- Agave – 2 tsp.
- Garlic powder - .5 tsp.
- Powdered ginger - .5 tsp.

**Mexican Marinade:**

- Light oil – 2 tbsp.
- Lime juice – 2 tbsp.
- Agave – 1 tbsp.
- Chili powder – 2 tsp.
- Smoked paprika – 1 tsp.
- Garlic powder - .5 tsp.

**Sweet and Smoky Marinade:**

- Olive oil – 2 tbsp.
- Maple syrup or agave – 2 tbsp.
- Soy sauce – 2 tbsp.
- Liquid smoke – 1 tsp.
- Garlic powder - .5 tsp.

- Chili powder - .5 tsp.

**Teriyaki Marinade:**

- Brown sugar – 2 tbsp.
- Soy sauce or substitute – 2 tbsp.
- Orange juice or water – 2 tbsp.
- Garlic powder - .5 tsp.
- Powdered ginger - .5 tsp.

**Instructions for the marinades:**

- For any marinade you choose, simply add all of the ingredients to a resealable bag or airtight container.
- Mix and add your <u>seitan tenders</u> or sliced/cubed tofu.
- Let them marinate for a minimum of 15 minutes or up to 4 days.

## Vegan Sour Cream

**Serving Yields**: Just over 1 cup

**Nutritional Counts**: Net Carbs: 1 g| Fat: 1 g

**Ingredients:**

- Extra-firm silken or crumbled firm tofu – 1 cup
- Rice milk – as needed – 2-3 tbsp.
- Lemon juice – 2 tsp. or to taste

- Salt - .25 tsp or as desired

**Preparation Method:**

- Mix all of the components in the blender or food processor. Puree until smooth.
- Store in an airtight container.

# Veggie Salsa

**Serving Yields**: 4

**Nutritional Counts**: Net Carbs: 4.9 g| Fat: 13.8 g

**Ingredients:**

- Cherry tomatoes – 2 cups
- Cucumber - 1
- Red onion - .5 of 1
- Lime juice - 2 tbsp.
- Chopped parsley - 2 tbsp.
- Garlic cloves - 2
- Extra-virgin olive oil - .25 cup
- Pepper and Salt – as desired

**Preparation Method:**

- Peel and dice the cucumber. Dice the rest of the veggies and mince the garlic.
- Toss all of the components into a serving dish. Enjoy as a side at your next party.

# Chapter 5: Appetizers – Sides and Snacks

## Sides

## Basil Zoodles and Olives

**Serving Yields**: 6

**Nutritional Counts**: Net Carbs: 8.4 g| Fat: 41.7 g

**Ingredients:**

- Fresh basil - .5 cup
- Spiralized zucchini – 4
- Avocado pesto - .5 cup
- Kalamata olives – 1 cup
- Drained sun-dried tomatoes - .25 cup
- Sliced avocados – 2
- Coconut oil – extra-virgin – 2 tbsp.
- Salt - .25 tsp.

**Preparation Method:**

- Remove the pits and drain the olives as you drain the tomatoes. Slice the avocados into strips.
- Spritz a pan with the coconut oil and prepare the noodles for two to five minutes – in batches if needed.
- Mix the pesto and noodles in a mixing container. Toss in the rest of the fixings and serve.

## Beetroot and Pesto Noodles

**Serving Yields**: 1

**Nutritional Counts**: Net Carbs: 13 g| Fat: 21 g

**Ingredients:**

- Beetroots - 2

**Pesto Ingredients:**

- Lime juice – 1 tsp.
- Avocado - 1
- Red chili pepper - 1
- Clove of garlic - 1

**Preparation Method:**

- Prepare the Fixings: Peel, spiralize, and lightly steam the beetroots. Peel and finely mince the garlic clove. Remove the seeds from the pepper and chop finely.
- Combine all of the pesto components.
- Toss the prepared noodles with the pesto and enjoy.

## Brussels Sprouts and Cashew Dip

**Serving Yields**: 10

**Nutritional Counts**: Net Carbs: 11.6g| Fat: 17 g

**Ingredients:**

- Trimmed Brussels sprouts – 1 lb.
- EVOO – 2 tbsp.
- Pepper - .25 tsp.
- Salt - .5 tsp.

**Ingredients for the dip:**

- Minced clove of garlic - 1
- Unsweetened Silk Cashew Milk – 1 cup
- Lemon juice – 3 tbsp.
- Unsweetened cashew butter – 1.5 cup
- Black pepper – 2 tsp.
- Coarse sea salt - .5 tsp.

**Preparation Method:**

- Set the oven temperature at 400°F.
- Toss the sprouts in a baking pan with the oil, pepper, and salt.
- Bake for 12-15 minutes. Set aside.
- Combine the dip fixings in a blender; mixing until smooth.
- Enjoy as a side dish at any time.

## Cabbage Slaw

**Serving Yields**: 2

**Nutritional Counts**: Net Carbs: 7 g| Fat: 33 g

**Ingredients:**

- Shredded green cabbage – 4 cups
- Tamari – 2 tbsp.
- Minced garlic cloves - 2
- Sesame oil – 1 tbsp.
- Vinegar – 1tsp.
- Chili paste – 1 tsp.
- Chopped Macadamia nuts - .5 cup

**Preparation Method:**

- Toss the fixings (omit the nuts) into a skillet using the low setting.
- Prepare covered for about 5 minutes. Stir in the nuts and continue cooking another five minutes.
- Serve and enjoy to complement any meal.

## Carrot and Zucchini Noodles in Thai Sauce

**Serving Yields**: 2

**Nutritional Counts**: Net Carbs: 9 g| Fat: 26 g

**Ingredients:**

- Carrot - 1
- Zucchini - 1
- Coconut milk - .5 cup
- Thai curry paste – 1 tbsp.

- Coconut oil – 2 tbsp.
- Also Needed: 1 Wok

**Preparation Method:**

- Peel and spiralize the carrot and zucchini.
- Warm up a wok and add the oil. Prepare the zucchini and carrots for 3-5 minutes.
- Combine the paste and milk. Stir in with the noodles.
- Continue to cook for another 30 seconds or so.

## Cauliflower and Artichoke Couscous

**Serving Yields**: 4

**Nutritional Counts:** Net Carbs: 8 g| Fat: 9 g

**Ingredients:**

- Black olives - 16
- Trimmed – riced - cauliflower head - 1
- Artichokes – 1 jar – 14 oz.
- Lemon – zest and juice - 1
- Olive oil – 2 tbsp.
- Black pepper and salt – .5 tsp.
- Parsley - .25 cup
- Clove of garlic - 1

**Preparation Method:**

- Finely chop the garlic and parsley after you trim the cauliflower head.
- Prepare a baking tray and toss it with the oil while adding the cauliflower.
- Bake at 400°F for 12 minutes. Toss about halfway through the cooking cycle.
- Fold in the rest of the fixings and enjoy.

## Cauliflower Bites with Ranch Dip

**Serving Yields**: 8

**Nutritional Counts**: Net Carbs: 2.4 g| Fat: 27.9 g

**Ingredients:**

- Cauliflower florets – 4 cups
- Garlic powder - .25 tsp.
- Salt - .25 tsp.
- Smoked paprika - .25 tsp.
- Extra-virgin olive oil – 2 tbsp.
- Sugar-free hot sauce - .5 cup

**Ingredients for the dip:**

- Unsweetened coconut milk - .5 cup
- Freshly squeezed lemon juice – 1 tbsp.
- Organic dairy-free mayo – 1 cup
- Garlic powder – 1 tsp.
- Pepper - .25 tsp.
- Onion powder – 1 tsp.

- Fresh parsley - .25 cup

**Preparation Method:**

- Whisk the ingredients for the dip and place in the fridge.
- Mix the hot sauce with the garlic powder, salt, and paprika. Toss in the cauliflower. Shake and then spread it in the prepared pan.
- Bake for 30 minutes.
- Serve with bites with the dip anytime you have a get-together with friends and family.

# Cherry Tomatoes and Zucchini Pasta

**Serving Yields**: 4

**Nutritional Counts**: Net Carbs: 13.1 g| Fat: 24 g

**Ingredients:**

- Thinly sliced red onion - 1
- Spiralized zucchini – 2 lb.
- Halved cherry tomatoes – 1 pint
- Minced cloves of garlic - 4
- Chopped basil - .5 cup
- EVOO - .25 cup
- Pepper and salt – as desired
- Crushed red pepper - .5 tsp.
- For the Topping: Shredded parmesan

**Preparation Method:**

- Warm up the oil in a pot. Sauté the garlic and onion. Toss in the zucchini, pepper, and salt. Cook 2 minutes, stirring once.

- Toss in the tomatoes and cook for 3-4 minutes. Then, add the basil and red pepper.

- Garnish with the cheese and serve.

## Chili and Coconut Cauliflower Rice

**Serving Yields**: 3

**Nutritional Counts**: Net Carbs: 4.6 g| Fat: 7.3 g

**Ingredients:**

- Full-fat coconut milk - .66 cup
- Riced cauliflower – 1 pkg.
- Onion powder - .5 tsp.
- Salt – as desired
- Chili paste – 1 tsp.
- Fresh basil – garnish

**Preparation Method:**

- Combine all of the components in a saucepan.
- Cook with the lid on for about 5-10 minutes. Stir every minute or so to prevent sticking.
- Take the lid off and continue cooking until it has absorbed the liquid.

# Coconut Cauliflower Rice

**Serving Yields**: 6

**Nutritional Counts**: Net Carbs: 3.1 g| Fat: 6.9 g

**Ingredients:**

- Full-fat coconut cream – 1 cup
- Chopped cauliflower - .5 of 1 head
- Cilantro – 1 tsp.
- Unsweetened shredded coconut - .25 cup
- Salt – to your liking

**Preparation Method:**

- Use a food processor to rice the cauliflower.
- Use the medium heat setting to warm a pan.
- Add all of the fixings and simmer until softened.
- Stir occasionally and serve when tender. It shouldn't take more than five minutes to prep and about ten minutes of cooking time for a delicious side dish.

# Creamy Curry Low-Carb Noodle Bowl

**Serving Yields**: 4

**Nutritional Counts**: Net Carbs: 7.3 g| Fat: 15.4 g

### Ingredients:

- Kanten Noodles – 1 pkg.
- Carrots – julienned - 2
- Cauliflower - roughly chopped - .5 of 1 head
- Red bell pepper - diced - 1
- Freshly chopped cilantro – 1 handful
- Mixed greens – 2 handfuls
- Dairy-free creamy curry sauce – 1 batch
- Water – Approx. 2 cups

### Preparation Method:

- Prepare the Kanten Noodles by placing the two sheets of noodles in a large bowl. Lightly heat the water, a couple of degrees below boiling. Think of it as hot water that you can drink.

- Pour water over the noodles and set aside while you prepare the rest of the ingredients. After about 5 minutes of soaking, strain and set aside in a large bowl to cool.

- Add carrots, cauliflower, bell pepper, and cilantro to the bowl with the noodles. Set mixed greens on 2 separate servings plates as the "base" to your meal.

- Then, prepare the Creamy Curry Sauce.

- Serve immediately or place in the fridge to cool for a couple of hours. Store in an air-tight container in the fridge for up to 2 days.

### For the creamy sauce:

**Serving Yields**: 4

**Nutritional Counts**: Net Carbs: 2.8 g| Fat: 15.2 g

### Ingredients:

- Avocado oil or MCT oil – 2 tbsp.
- Tahini or avocado oil mayo - .25 cup
- Water - .25 cup

- Apple cider vinegar – 2 tbsp.
- Ground coriander – 1.5 tsp.
- Curry powder - 2 tsp.
- Sea salt – 1 tsp.
- Freshly-cracked black pepper - .5 tsp.
- Turmeric – 1 tsp.
- Cumin – 1 tsp.
- Ground ginger - .25 tsp.

**Preparation Method:**
- Combine all of the fixings into the jug of a high-powered blender.
- Pulse until smooth.
- Add the veggie and noodle mixture and toss to coat.

## Edamame Kelp Noodles

**Serving Yields**: 2

**Nutritional Counts**: Net Carbs: 4.9 g| Fat: 8.6 g

**Ingredients:**

- Kelp noodles – 1 pkg.
- Frozen spinach – 1 cup
- Shelled edamame - .5 cup
- Julienned carrots - .25 cup
- Sliced mushrooms - .25 cup

**Ingredients for the sauce:**

- Sesame oil - 1 tbsp.
- Tamari – 2 tbsp.

- Garlic powder - .5 tsp.
- Ground ginger - .5 tsp.
- Sriracha - .25 tsp.

**Preparation Method:**
- Prepare the noodles in a pan of water to soak. Drain well.
- Combine the sauce components in a pan using the medium heat setting.
- Toss in the vegetables.
- Once the mixture is hot, toss in the soaked noodles.
- Simmer and stir occasionally with a lid on until steamy hot.

## Garlicky Mushrooms

**Serving Yields**: 3

**Nutritional Counts**: Net Carbs: 5 g| Fat: 8 g

**Ingredients for Step # 1:**
- Minced garlic cloves - 4
- Cremini mushrooms - 24 oz.
- Bay leaves - 2
- Dried oregano - .5 tsp.
- Dried basil - .5 tsp.
- Dried thyme - .25 tsp.
- Vegetable broth – 1 cup

- Black pepper and salt – to your liking
- Unsalted butter – 2 tbsp.
- Half and Half - .25 cup
- Parsley – 2 tbsp.

**Preparation Method:**

- Mix all of the fixings (step 1) in a slow cooker and prepare using the low setting for 3-4 hours.
- About 20 minutes before it's done; combine the butter and Half and Half for the sauce.
- Garnish with freshly chopped parsley and enjoy.

## Grilled Eggplant and Zucchini

**Serving Yields**: 2

**Nutritional Counts**: Net Carbs: 6 g| Fat: 14 g

**Ingredients:**

- Eggplants - 2
- Zucchinis - 2
- Garlic cloves - 2
- Parsley - 2 tbsp.
- Mint - 2 tbsp.
- Olive oil – 4 tsp.
- Erythritol – 1 tbsp.
- Red wine vinegar – 4 tsp.

- Pepper and salt – to taste

**Preparation Method:**

- Slice the zucchini and eggplants lengthwise. Chop the veggies.
- Brush the eggplant and zucchini with the oil. Sprinkle with the salt and pepper.
- Place on a hot griddle pan and brown on both sides. Place on the serving dish.
- Warm up the rest of the oil and sauté the garlic. Add the erythritol and vinegar. Pour over the veggies and garnish with the mint and parsley.

## Indian Curried Cauliflower

**Serving Yields**: 4

**Nutritional Counts**: Net Carbs: 5 g| Fat: 7 g

**Ingredients:**

- Peanut oil – 2 tbsp.
- Cauliflower - .5 of 1 head - chopped
- Cumin seeds – 1 tsp.
- Chopped shallots - .5 cup
- Pepper and salt -to taste
- Sweet curry – 1.5 tsp.
- Chopped cilantro - .25 cup
- Lime – juiced - 1

**Preparation Method:**

- Warm up a 'wide' pan and sauté the seeds for about 30 seconds.

- Toss in the shallots, cauliflower, pepper, salt, and curry powder. Cook for 7-8 minutes – stirring occasionally.
- Toss in the cilantro. Serve with a drizzle of the lime juice.

## Kelp Noodles with Peanut Butter Sauce

**Serving Yields**: 4

**Nutritional Counts**: Net Carbs: 2 g| Fat: 16 g

**Ingredients:**
- Kelp Noodles
- White onion – 1
- Garlic cloves – 3
- Peanut butter - .5 cup
- Soy sauce – keto-friendly - .25 cup
- Lime juiced – 1
- Red pepper flakes – 2 tsp.

**Preparation Method:**
- Soak the kelp noodles in water and drain.
- Combine all of the sauce fixings in a blender. Mix well until creamy.
- When ready to serve, just add the sauce on the top of the noodles. Enjoy.

## Lime and Chili Carrot Noodles

**Serving Yields**: 1

**Nutritional Counts:** Net Carbs: 4 g| Fat: 27 g

### Ingredients:

- Jalapeno chilis - 2
- Carrots - 2
- Lime juice - 1 tbsp.
- Coconut oil - 2 tbsp.
- Coriander - .25 cup
- Black pepper - .5 tsp.
- Salt - .5 tsp.

### Preparation Method:

- Prepare the vegetables. Deseed and finely chop the jalapenos. Peel and spiralize the carrots and finely chop the coriander.
- Combine the oil, lime juice, and jalapeno. Toss and add the carrots.
- Blend in the rest of the fixings and serve.

## Mediterranean Spaghetti Squash

**Serving Yields:** 4

**Nutritional Counts:** Net Carbs: 14.77 g| Fat: 22.91 g

### Ingredients:

- Spaghetti squash - 1
- Pine nuts – 2 tbsp.
- Pesto - .25 cup

- Kalamata olives - .33 cup
- Freshly chopped basil - .25 cup
- Cherry tomatoes - 10
- Cremini mushrooms – 10 oz.
- Salt and pepper – as desired
- Olive oil – as needed

**Preparation Method:**

- Set the oven temperature to 400°F. Cover a baking sheet with parchment paper.
- Slice the squash -lengthwise- and remove the seeds. Drizzle with the oil, pepper, and salt. Place in the pan (cut side down) and bake 30-40 minutes. Let it rest for about 10 minutes.
- Meanwhile, add the mushrooms to a parchment paper-lined pan. Give them a splatter of oil, salt, and pepper. Bake until browning begins (10-15 min.).
- Using the medium heat setting to combine the pesto and squash in a large skillet. Cook for 3-4 minutes until the squash is slightly crispy.
- Lower the heat (medium) and add the rest of the fixings. Cook for another 5-10 minutes; stir frequently and season to your liking.

## Mushroom, Broccoli, and Squash Noodles

**Serving Yields**: 1

**Nutritional Counts**: Net Carbs: 5.4 g| Fat: 17.51 g

**Ingredients:**

- Broccoli florets - .5 cup
- Spiralized summer squash - 1

- Chopped almonds - 5
- Halved cherry tomatoes - 5
- Olive oil – 1 tbsp.
- Sliced cremini mushrooms - 5
- Parsley pesto – 2 tbsp.

**Preparation Method:**

- Warm up a skillet with the oil. When hot, toss in the mushrooms. Add the florets of broccoli and stir about 2 minutes (half cooked).
- Add the squash 'noodles' and stir for another 2 minutes.
- Transfer to the countertop and add the rest of the fixings.

## Nutty Pesto Zucchini

**Serving Yields**: 2

**Nutritional Counts**: Net Carbs: 11.46 g| Fat: 26.08 g

### Ingredients:

- Basil leaves - 5
- Zucchinis – ribbon slices - 3
- Salt - .5 tsp.
- Olive oil – 1 tbsp.
- Parmesan cheese - .25 cup

### Ingredients for the Pesto:

- Walnuts - .25 cup

- Peeled garlic cloves - 2
- Avocado - .5 of 1
- Water – if necessary - .5 of a cup
- Fresh basil leaves – 1 cup
- Lemon - .5 of 1

**Preparation Method:**

- After slicing the zucchini, sprinkle it with the salt, and set aside for now.
- Use a blender and add the pesto components – blending until smooth. Add water if needed.
- Warm up the oil in a pan and simmer the zucchini for 4 minutes.
- Transfer to a platter with the pesto. Sprinkle with the cheese and basil before serving.

## Pesto Kelp Noodles

**Serving Yields**: 3

**Nutritional Counts**: Net Carbs: 1.3 g| Fat: 32.7 g

**Ingredients:**

- Kelp noodles – 1 pkg.

**Pesto Ingredients:**

- Baby spinach leaves – 1 cup
- Haas avocado – 1 pitted
- Cloves of garlic - 2

- EVOO - .5 cup
- Basil - .25 cup
- Salt – 1 tsp.

**Preparation Method:**

- Rinse and soak the noodles for about 30 minutes.
- Mix the pesto fixings in a blender until creamy smooth.
- Drain and toss the noodles into about ¼ cup of the sauce. Save the rest for another time!

## Roasted Beetroot Noodles

**Serving Yields**: 3

**Nutritional Counts:** Net Carbs: 10 g| Fat: 25 g

**Ingredients:**

- Baby kale – 2 cups
- Spiralized beets - 2

**Ingredients for the Pesto:**

- Pine nuts - .25 cup
- Olive oil - .25 cup
- Basil leaves – 3 cups
- Ground black pepper - .5 tsp.
- Ground sea salt - .5 tsp.
- Minced garlic clove - 1

**Preparation Method:**

- Prepare a baking tin with a layer of non-stick cooking spray.
- After spiralizing the noodles, give them a dusting of the pepper and salt.
- Heat up the oven to 425°F. Prepare for 5 minutes or to your liking.
- Combine the pesto fixings in a food processor until smooth.
- Toss it all together and enjoy.

## Roasted Broccoli

**Serving Yields**: 4

**Nutritional Counts**: Net Carbs: 7 g| Fat: 14.3 g

**Ingredients:**

- Extra-virgin olive oil - .25 cup
- Broccoli – 2 - into florets
- Salt - .5 tsp.
- Minced garlic cloves - 2

**Preparation Method:**

- Incorporate all of the fixings and add to a baking dish.
- Set the oven temperature to reach 450°F. When hot, add the prepared veggies to the oven and bake for 15 minutes.
- Serve for a luncheon treat or dinner side dish.
- 

## Roasted Green Cabbage

**Serving Yields**: 2

**Nutritional Counts**: Net Carbs: 9 g| Fat: 21 g

**Ingredients:**

- Green cabbage head - 1
- Garlic cloves - 4
- Olive oil – 4 tbsp.
- Pepper and salt – as desired

**Preparation Method:**

- Peel and mince the garlic cloves. Remove the outer leaves of the cabbage and slice the remainder into 6-inch slices. Add the slices to a baking sheet.

- Brush the fixings with oil and about half of the garlic. Give it a sprinkle of salt and pepper.
- Set the oven to 400°F. Prepare for 20 minutes. Flip the cabbage and sprinkle with the rest of the garlic. Continue baking for 20 more minutes.
- Serve piping hot!

## Roasted Kale and Squash

**Serving Yields**: 8

**Nutritional Counts**: Net Carbs: 10 g| Fat: 35 g

### Ingredients:

- Torn kale – 2 tbsp.
- Spaghetti squash – 1
- Chili powder - .5 tsp.
- Pepper and salt- to taste
- Balsamic vinegar – 1 tsp.
- Diced onion - .5 of 1
- Olive oil – as needed

### Preparation Method:

- Remove the seeds and cut the squash into halves. Place it cut side up on a baking sheet. Cover it with some of the oil.
- Prepare the oven setting to 350°F. Bake until done.
- Meanwhile, add 1 tbsp. of oil to a skillet and sauté the onion for about 3 minutes. Add to the kale with a shake of salt and pepper. Bake for another 5 minutes.

- Remove the squash strands and add the vinegar, a tbsp. of oil, and the chili powder. Serve together and enjoy.

## Spaghetti Squash

**Serving Yields**: 4

**Nutritional Counts**: Net Carbs: 4 g| Fat: 7 g

**Ingredients:**

- 
- Olive oil – 2 tbsp.
- Spaghetti squash 1 whole
- Sage - .5 tsp.
- Cracked pepper - .5 tsp.
- Salt – 1 tsp.
- Dried parsley – 1 tsp.
- Garlic powder – 1 tsp.
- Dried rosemary – 1 tsp.
- Dried thyme – 1 tsp.
- Also needed: Baking pan

**Preparation Method:**

- Set the oven temperature to 350°F.
- Cut the squash in half and discard the seeds. Add some water to the baking tin and add the squash – cut side downwards.

- Roast for 45 minutes to 1 hour.
- Remove and cool. Scoop out all of the flesh and add to a mixing bowl with the rest of the fixings.
- Cook for another 15 minutes before serving.

## Sriracha Grilled Asparagus

**Serving Yields**: 4

**Nutritional Counts**: Net Carbs: 3.75 g| Fat: 17 g

### Ingredients:

- Trimmed asparagus – 1 lb.
- Kosher salt - to taste
- Olive oil – 1 tsp.

### Ingredients for the sauce:

- Avocado oil - .25 cup
- Sriracha sauce - 1 tbsp.
- Lime juice - 1 tbsp.
- Vegan-friendly tamari – 2 tsp
- Rice wine vinegar – 2 tbsp.
- Granulated sugar-free sweetener – your choice – 1 tsp.

### Preparation Method:

- Toss the salt, oil, and asparagus together. Place on the grill and cook until tender.
- Prepare the sauce. Whisk the fixings (not the pecans). Then, blend in the pecans.

- Pour the sauce over the grilled asparagus and serve to your waiting guests.

## Teriyaki Grilled Eggplant

**Serving Yields**: 5

**Nutritional Counts**: Net Carbs: 6.98 g| Fat:12.07 g

**Ingredients:**

- Cloves of garlic - 2
- Medium eggplants - 2
- Sesame oil - .25 cup
- Liquid aminos - .5 cup
- Ground ginger – 1 tbsp.
- Granulated swerve – 2 tbsp.
- Toasted sesame seeds – 1 tbsp.

**Preparation Method:**

- Peel and crush the garlic cloves. Use the medium heat setting and combine the garlic, sesame oil, liquid aminos, swerve, and ginger into a saucepan.

- Once it is gently simmering, continue frequently stirring until it begins to thicken slightly. Take it off of the burner and set aside for now.

- Warm up the grill. Remove the stems from the eggplants. Cut into slices about 1/8-inch thick. Brush each eggplant slice with the teriyaki sauce and place on the grill.

- Sear each side, brushing with more sauce as it caramelizes. Top it off with a portion of the sauce and some toasted sesame seeds.

## Tofu Pizza Sticks

**Serving Yields**: 4

**Nutritional Counts**: Net Carbs: 3.8 g| Fat: 5.7 g

**Ingredients:**

- Extra-firm tofu – 1 block
- Tomato sauce - .25 cup (+) 1 tbsp.
- Nutritional yeast – 2 tbsp. (+) 2 tsp.
- Dried basil – 1-2 pinches

**Preparation Method:**

- Drain the Tofu: Wrap the block of tofu in a paper towel. Weigh down something heavy on top to press. Let the tofu drain for about 15-20 minutes.
- Warm up the oven to reach 425°F. Prepare a cookie sheet with a layer of parchment paper.
- Slice the tofu into 16 thin pieces and arrange in the pan. Spread the sauce on each of the sticks. Sprinkle with the nutritional yeast and a dusting of the basil to taste.
- Bake for 27-30 minutes

## Turnip Fries

**Serving Yields**: 6

**Nutritional Counts**: Net Carbs: 4.4 g| Fat: 9.5 g

**Ingredients:**

- Organic turnips – 2 lb.
- Taco seasoning – 2 tbsp.
- Unrefined sea salt - .5 tsp.
- Light olive oil - .25 cup

**Preparation Method:**

- Set the oven temperature at 350°F.
- Peel and chop the turnips (chip-thin). Combine all of the fixings in a Ziploc-type baggie and shake well.
- Prepare a baking tin with parchment paper and add the fries.
- Bake until golden – tossing about halfway through (25 min.).

## Turnip and Courgette Hash Browns

**Serving Yields**: 1

**Nutritional Counts**: Net Carbs: 8 g| Fat: 12 g

**Ingredients:**

- Courgetti – grated with moisture removed - .5 cup
- Grated turnip – 1 cup
- Grated onion – 1
- Garlic powder – 1 tsp.
- Pepper and salt – to taste
- Olive oil – 2 tbsp.
- Fresh thyme – 1 tbsp.

**Preparation Method:**

- Combine all of the fixings except for the olive oil.
- Warm up the oil in a skillet. Toss in small portions of the mixture.
- Simmer until golden brown and flip. Finish cooking the second side.
- Continue until done and serve.

## Zucchini Noodles and Avocado Sauce

**Serving Yields**: 2

**Nutritional Counts**: Net Carbs: 9 g| Fat: 26.8 g

**Ingredients:**

- Zucchini - 1
- Basil - 1.25 cups
- Water - .33 cup
- Avocado - 1
- Pine nuts – 4 tbsp.
- Sliced cherry tomatoes - 12
- Lemon juice – 2 tbsp.

**Preparation Method:**

- Use a spiralizer or a veggie peeler to prepare the zucchini noodles.
- Combine the remainder of the fixings (except the tomatoes) in a blender until creamy smooth.
- Mix together the avocado sauce, noodles, and cherry tomatoes in a mixing container.

- You can enjoy these delicious noodles stored in the refrigerator for one or two days.

# Snack Time Treats

## Carrot Cake Bites

**Serving Yields**: 15

**Nutritional Counts**: Net Carbs: 1 g| Fat: 1 g

**Ingredients:**

- Coconut flour - .5 cup
- Water - .5 cup (+) 1 tbsp.
- Unsweetened applesauce – 2 tbsp.
- Vanilla extract - .5 tsp.
- Cinnamon – 1 tsp.
- Granulated Lakanto Monk Fruit Sweetener HYPERLINK "https://www.lakanto.com/collections/display-products/products/lakanto-classic-sugar-free-sweetener-family-size-800g?aff=6" - 4 tbsp.
- Carrot - 1 medium
- Reduced fat shredded coconut – 4 tbsp.

**Preparation Method:**

- Combine the coconut flour, applesauce, water, and vanilla extract in a large mixing bowl. Stir well.
- Finely shred or chop the carrot. Add in cinnamon, Lakanto, and shredded carrots to a bowl, and stir to combine. Refrigerate dough for 15 minutes.
- Place the shredded coconut in small bowl.
- After 15 minutes, remove dough from fridge and roll into 15 cake balls. Roll each ball in shredded coconut until evenly coated.
- Store in refrigerator for up to a week.

- Tip: You can use another granulated sweetener of choice, equivalent to 4 tablespoons of sugar.

## Chocolate Granola

**Serving Yields**: 32

**Nutritional Counts**: Net Carbs: 4.2 g| Fat: 17.5 g

**Ingredients:**

- 
- Unsweetened cocoa - .125 cup
- Melted coconut oil – 1.8 oz.
- Granulated sweetener – your favorite – 2 tbsp.
- Cinnamon – 1 tsp.
- Pumpkin seeds – 3.5 oz.
- Shredded coconut – 3.5 oz.
- Sunflower seeds – 3.5 oz.
- Chopped almonds – 3.5 oz.
- Flaxseeds – 3.5 oz.
- Chopped walnuts – 3.5 oz.

**Preparation Method:**

- Warm the oven to reach 350°F.
- Combine the sweetener, cinnamon, coconut oil, and cocoa.

- Toss the seeds, coconut, and all of the nuts in a baking dish and add the mixture from (step 2). Stir well.

- Bake for 20 minutes until browned and crispy. Toss every 4 minutes.

## Chocolate Protein Bars

**Serving Yields**: 8

**Nutritional Counts**: Net Carbs: 1.4 g| Fat: 13.9 g

**Ingredients:**

- Raw hemp hearts - .75 cup
- Raw sunflower seeds - .5 cup
- Cocoa powder - .25 cup
- Chia seeds - .25 cup
- Psyllium husk powder – 2 tbsp.
- Salt - .5 tsp.
- Liquid stevia - .25 tsp.
- Water – 1 cup

**Preparation Method:**

- Preheat the oven temperature to 250°F.
- Grind the seeds to a flour-like texture. Combine with the dry fixings.
- Add the water – as you stir- to form a thick dough. Spread the batter on a baking sheet to a 1-inch thickness.
- Bake for 1 1/2 hours.
- Divide the bars into eight servings and bake for another 15 minutes.

- Serve or enjoy anytime.

## Cinnamon Granola

**Serving Yields**: 4

**Nutritional Counts**: Net Carbs: 3.74 g| Fat: 19.08 g

**Ingredients:**

- Unsweetened coconut flakes - 5 tbsp.
- Ground flax meal - 5 tbsp.
- Chia seeds – 1 tbsp.
- Sugar-free maple syrup – 4 tbsp.
- Nuts – walnuts, pecans, etc. – 1.5 oz.
- Cinnamon – 1.5 tsp.

**Preparation Method:**

- Prepare a baking sheet with a layer of baking parchment paper. Heat the oven to 350°F.
- Combine everything (omit the cinnamon) in a mixing bowl.
- Mix well and spread out over the baking tin with a sprinkle of the cinnamon– single layer.
- Bake, stirring once, for 20-22 minutes.
- Remove and let the granola harden. Store using an airtight bowl.

## Coconut and Peanut Butter Balls

**Serving Yields**: 15

**Nutritional Counts**: Net Carbs: 0.92 g| Fat: 3.19 g

### Ingredients:

- Unsweetened coconut powder – 3 tsp.
- Creamy peanut butter – vegan-friendly – 3 tbsp.
- Almond flour – 2 tsp.
- Powdered erythritol – 2.5 tsp.
- Coconut flakes - .5 cup

### Preparation Method:

- Combine the cocoa, flour, peanut butter, and erythritol. Mix well and freeze 1 hour. Use a small spoon to scoop out the mixture.
- Drop it into the flakes of coconut. Roll it around with your hand and refrigerate overnight for the best firming results.

## Fudge Balls

**Serving Yields**: 12

**Nutritional Counts**: Net Carbs: 7.4 g| Fat: 28.8 g

### Ingredients:

- Unsweetened cocoa powder - .5 cup
- Almond, peanut, or cashew nut butter – 1 cup
- Coconut oil – 1 cup
- Coconut flour - .33 cup

- Pink Himalayan salt – 1 pinch
- Monk fruit sweetener - .5 to 1 tsp. or .25 tsp. powdered stevia

**Preparation Method:**

- Combine the chosen nut butter and add it and the coconut oil in a saucepan (med. heat). Stir in the rest of the fixings.
- Freeze in a glass dish for 20 minutes until it's firmed up somewhat.
- Remove and form into 1-inch balls. You must work quickly, or the oil will melt.
- Return to the freezer for 10-15 minutes. Store in a closed container in the freezer.

## Loaded Nut-Packed Coconut Granola

**Serving Yields:** 20

**Nutritional Counts:** Net Carbs: 5.9 g| Fat: 18.5 g

**Ingredients:**

- Unsweetened coconut flakes - .5 cup
- Raw pecans – 1.25 cups
- Raw walnuts – 1 cup
- Raw almonds – 2 cups
- Chia seeds - 3 tbsp.
- Ground cinnamon – 1.5 tsp.
- Sea salt - .25 tsp.
- Flaxseed meal – 1 tbsp.
- Coconut sugar – 2 tbsp.
- Maple syrup - .25 cup (+) 1 tbsp.

- Coconut oil - 3 tbsp.
- Roasted – unsalted – Sunflower seeds - .25 cup
- Dried blueberries - .25 cup

**Preparation Method:**

- Prepare the oven temperature to 325°F.
- Combine the coconut sugar, nuts, coconut, flaxseed meal, salt, and cinnamon in a mixing container.
- Warm up the maple syrup and coconut oil using the medium heat setting (stovetop). Pour into the mixture (Step 1).
- Add the fixings to the baking sheet and spread as evenly as possible.
- Bake in the preheated oven for 20 minutes.
- Transfer to the countertop. Stir in the blueberries and sunflower seeds.
- Bake for another 5-8 minutes at 340°F.
- Transfer from the oven and set on a cooling rack to cool.

## Mushroom Chips

**Serving Yields**: 4

**Nutritional Counts**: Net Carbs: 3.8 g| Fat: 15.5g

### Ingredients:

- Coconut oil – 4 tbsp.
- Portobello mushrooms – 10.6 oz.
- Salt - .5 tsp.
- Dash- Ground black pepper

### Preparation Method:

- Brush a little oil on the baking sheet.
- Slice the mushrooms thin and add to the prepared tin.
- Sprinkle with the pepper and salt and bake at 300°F for 45-60 minutes.
- Flip 2-3 times during the process for even browning.

# Pecan and Maple Fat Bars

**Serving Yields**: 12

**Nutritional Counts**: Net Carbs: 2 g| Fat: 30.5 g

## Ingredients:

- Halved pecans – 2 cups
- Almond flour – 1 cup
- Golden flaxseed meal - .5 cup
- Shredded coconut – unsweetened - .5 cup
- Coconut oil - .5 cup
- Liquid stevia - .25 tsp.
- Maple syrup – keto friendly - .25 cup

## Preparation Method:

- Program the oven setting to 350°F. Add the pecans to a pan and toast 6-7 minutes. Cool and crush in a plastic bag.
- Combine all of the dry components – including the pecans. Stir in the wet ingredients to form a crumbly dough. Spread it onto a baking dish and press. Prepare in the hot oven for 20-15 minutes.
- Take the bars out of the oven to cool for 15-20 minutes. Next, place in the fridge for about 1 hour until cold.
- Serve and enjoy any time.

# Peanut Butter Fat Bombs

**Serving Yields**: 24

**Nutritional Counts**: Net Carbs: 2.4 g| Fat: 8.7 g

**Ingredients:**

- Extra-virgin coconut oil - .5 cup
- Peanut Butter - smooth style, with salt -- sugar-free - .5 cup
- Trader Joes Coco Powder unsweetened 3 serving or 1 tbsp.
- Vanilla extract - .5 tsp
- Pyure Organic Stevia all-purpose sweetener - 9 tsp.
- NOW MCT Oil – 2 tbsp.
- Jif Powdered Peanut Butter - 2 tbsp.

**Preparation Method:**

- Melt your coconut oil and your peanut butter. Then, mix using a hand mixer. Next, add the coco powder and your vanilla. Mix - scraping the sides as needed.

- For the Pyure, you will want to adjust to your sweetness liking. It will need to be ground in a coffee grinder to give it a powdered sugar texture.

  Then pour it into the bowl. Mix well and add the powdered PB and the CT and mix again.

- Pour into ice cube tray and store in the freezer compartment of the fridge until set for about one hour. Then, you can store them in the fridge in a container. Use parchment paper to separate layers if you stack them.

## Peanut Tofu Wrap

**Serving Yields**: 4

**Nutritional Counts**: Net Carbs: 5 g| Fat: 12 g

**Ingredients:**

- Crumbled extra-firm tofu – 1 pkg. 16 oz.
- Savoy cabbage leaves - 4 Large
- Canola oil – 1 tbsp.
- Prepared peanut sauce – 5 tbsp.
- Salt - .25 tsp.
- Rice vinegar – 1 tbsp.
- Julienned Asian pear – 1 cup
- Lime zest – 1.5 tsp.
- Julienned English cucumber – 1 cup
- Cilantro – finely chopped - .25 cup

**Preparation Method:**

- Cut the cabbage crosswise and into halves. Crumble the tofu.
- Warm up a skillet and add the oil. Sauté the tofu for 4-6 minutes (seasoned with salt) until lightly browned.
- Whisk the peanut sauce, vinegar, and zested lime. Take the pan from the burner and mix the sauce. Toss well.
- Add the tofu fixings to each of the cabbage pieces.
- Garnish with the cilantro, pear, and cucumber. Serve.

## Roasted Radish Chips

**Serving Yields:** 4

**Nutritional Counts:** Net Carbs: 1.2 g| Fat: 7.1 g

### Ingredients:

- Radishes – 16 oz.
- Pepper and salt - .5 tsp. of ea.
- Coconut oil – 2 tbsp.

### Preparation Method:

- Chop the radishes into thin rounds. Toss all of the fixings together.
- Bake – single-layered – at 400°F for 12-15 minutes.
- Enjoy for a quick and tasty treat anytime.

## Sweet Potato Toast

**Serving Yields**: 4

**Nutritional Counts**: Net Carbs: 9.02 g| Fat: 23.85 g

### Ingredients:

- Ripe avocado - 1
- Large sweet potato - 1
- Pepper and salt – as desired
- Roughly-chopped pistachios - .5 cup
- Olive oil – 3 tbsp.
- Crushed red pepper flakes - optional

### Preparation Method:

- Warm up the oven to 400°F. Prepare a baking sheet with aluminum foil.

- Slice the potato into 1/4-inch rounds. Arrange on the baking sheet and toss it with the oil, salt, and pepper.
- Bake for 20 minutes and garnish with the avocado and pistachios. Add a few pepper flakes.

## Zucchini Chips

**Serving Yields**: 8

**Nutritional Counts**: Net Carbs: 2.3 g| Fat: 3.6 g

**Ingredients:**

- Zucchini – 4 cups
- Coarse sea salt – 2 tsp.
- EVOO – 2 tbsp.
- White balsamic vinegar – 2 tbsp.

**Preparation Method:**

- Cover a baking pan with parchment paper.
- Thinly slice the zucchini. Whisk the oil and vinegar together and toss with the zucchini.
- Arrange the zucchini on the baking tin in an even layer. Give it a sprinkle of salt.
- Bake at 200°F for 2-3 hours. Flip about halfway through the cooking process. Enjoy any time.

# Chapter 6: Desserts – Smoothies and Beverages

## Pudding Specialties

### Avocado and Chocolate Pudding

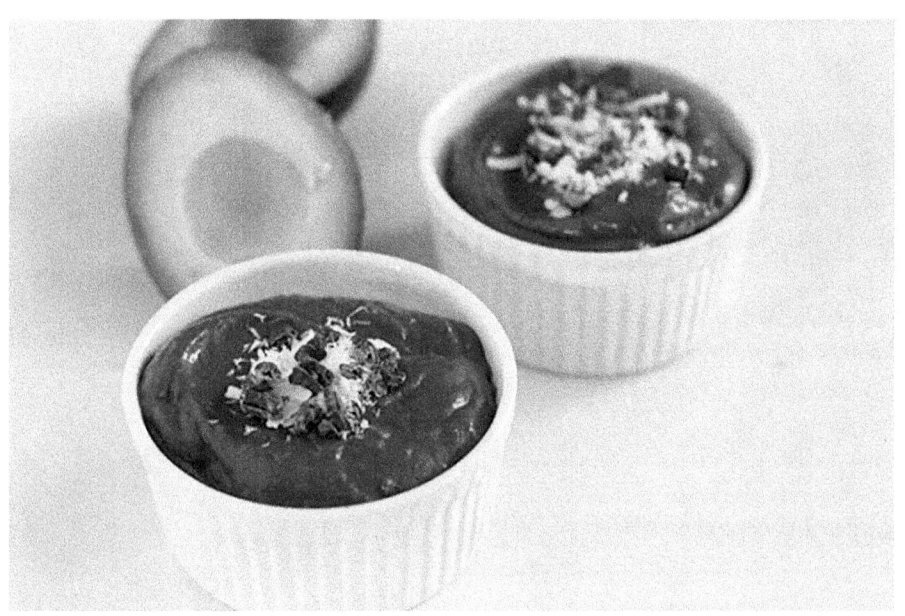

**Serving Yields**: 1

**Nutritional Counts**: Net Carbs: 6 g| Fat: 24 g

**Ingredients:**

- Avocado – pit removed - 1
- Cocoa powder - .25 cup
- Pink salt – 1 tsp.
- Vanilla extract - .5 tsp.
- Stevia – 10 drops

**Preparation Method:**

- Combine the fixings in a mixing bowl. Beat well with a fork. Continue whipping until it is as you like it!

- Chill and serve.

## Chia Chocolate Pudding

**Serving Yields**: 8

**Nutritional Counts**: Net Carbs: 14.9 g| Fat: 16.5 g

**Ingredients for Day 1:**
- Vanilla extract – 1 tsp.
- Coconut milk – 2 cups
- Unsweetened cocoa powder - .25 cup
- Maple syrup - .25 cup
- Salt – 1 pinch
- Chia seeds - .66 cup

**Ingredients for Day 2:**
- Unsweetened shredded coconut - 1 tbsp.
- Coconut milk- 1 tbsp.
- Optional: Whipped cream - 1 tbsp.
- Coconut sugar – 1 tsp.

**Preparation Method:**

- Day 1 Prep: Whisk all of Day 1's ingredients, adding the chia seeds last. Add the mixture to a large jar with a lid to combine for about five minutes.
- Gently rotate the jar for 30 seconds and rest for four minutes. Continue for 20 more minutes. Place the mixture in the fridge overnight or at least for eight hours.
- Day 2 Prep: Add the pudding into a mixing container and blend the ingredients (omit the milk).
- Drizzle with 1 tbsp. of coconut milk over the top of the pudding.
- Garnish as desired.

## Chia Raspberry Pudding

**Serving Yields**: 4

**Nutritional Counts**: Net Carbs: 4.3 g| Fat: 18.2 g

**Ingredients:**

- Coconut milk – 1 cup
- Water - .5 cup
- Fresh raspberries – 1 cup
- Whole chia seeds - .5 cup
- Vanilla powder – 1 tsp.

**Preparation Method:**

- Mix the raspberries, milk, and water in a blender until smooth.
- Fold in the chia seeds and vanilla.
- Chill the pudding overnight for best results.

# Chia Strawberry Pudding

**Serving Yields**: 1

**Nutritional Counts**: Net Carbs: 11 g| Fat: 57 g

### Ingredients:

- Stevia – 1 dash
- Chopped strawberries - .25 cup
- Chia seeds – 2 tbsp.
- Vanilla essence - .5 tsp.
- Coconut milk – 1 cup

### Preparation Method:

- Combine the ingredients in a canning jar with a lid. Close the top and shake well.
- Store in the refrigerator for at least eight hours. Enjoy this treat anytime!

# Coconut Chia and Turmeric Pudding

**Serving Yields**: 1

**Nutritional Counts**: Net Carbs: 14 g| Fat: 78 g

### Ingredients:

- Chia seeds – 2 tbsp.
- Coconut milk – 6 oz.

- Ground cardamom - .25 tsp.
- Unsweetened desiccated coconut - .5 cup
- Peeled and grated turmeric – 1 piece – 1-inch
- Also Needed: 1 mason jar

**Preparation Method:**
- Mix all of the fixings in a mason jar and close the top.
- Shake the jar to mix well and let the goodies steep overnight in the fridge.
- Wake up to a ready-to-go meal for one of those fast-moving mornings.

## Pumpkin and Peanut Butter Pudding

**Serving Yields**: 2

**Nutritional Counts**: Net Carbs: 13 g| Fat: 61 g

**Ingredients:**
- Pumpkin puree - .5 cup
- Peanut Butter – keto-friendly - .5 cup
- Chia seeds – 2 tbsp.
- Coconut milk – 1 cup

**Preparation Method:**
- Measure out and all of the fixings into a blender.
- Give the container a quick blitz and pour into a mason jar.

- Place in the fridge to chill; overnight preferably.

## Other Delicious Desserts

### Avocado Chocolate Mousse

**Serving Yields**: 3 generous portions

**Nutritional Counts**: Net Carbs: 19 g| Fat: 27 g

**Ingredients:**

- Chopped semisweet chocolate – 4 oz. *or* at least 60% dark chocolate chips – or about .5 cup (+) 2 tbsp.

- Large ripe avocados - 2 - 8 oz. ea.

- Kosher salt - .125 tsp.

- Unsweetened cocoa powder – 3 tbsp.

- Unsweetened <u>Almond Breeze Blend</u> - .25 cup

- Pure vanilla extract – 1 tsp.

- Optional: Light agave nectar 1–3 tsp. - pure maple syrup

- For Serving: Sliced strawberries or fresh raspberries - whipped coconut cream, and a few chocolate shavings

**Preparation Method:**

- Use a microwave-safe and toss in the chips of chocolate. Melt for 15 seconds at a time, mixing well. Stir well and set aside to cool.

- Slice the avocado and remove the pit. Add to a food processor along with the cocoa powder, salt, melted chocolate, milk blend, and vanilla extract. Continue blending scraping the sides until creamy smooth.

- Adjust the sweetness with a few teaspoons of the agave as desired.

- Spoon into glasses and enjoy immediately as a pudding or for a thicker, mousse-like consistency. For best results, chill overnight or a minimum of two hours.

- Serve topped with raspberries, cream, and chocolate shavings.

## Banana Bread

**Serving Yields**: 12

**Nutritional Counts**: Net Carbs: 4 g| Fat: 8 g

**Ingredients:**

- Blanched almond flour – 2 cups
- Granulated sweetener of choice – 2 tbsp.
- Cinnamon - 1 tsp.
- Baking powder – 1 tsp.
- Salt - .25 tsp.
- Large overripe bananas, mashed – 2
- Flax eggs –2 - replacement for 2 regular hen eggs
- Coconut oil - .5 cup
- Vanilla extract – 1 tsp.

**Preparation Method:**

- Warm up the oven to reach 350°F. Grease a loaf pan or 10 x 10-inch square pan and set to the side.

- Combine the dry fixings in a mixing container, mixing well. In a separate bowl, melt your coconut oil. Add your mashed bananas and flax eggs/eggs and whisk together.

- Combine all of the fixings (dry and wet) and toss until entirely incorporated. Pour into the greased pan. Bake for 40-50 minutes.

- Note: A square pan tends to be around the 40-minute mark, whereas a loaf pan is at the 45-50-minute mark or until a toothpick comes out clean from the center.

- Cool the cake in the pan for ten minutes. Then, move it to cool onto a wire rack. Slice and serve.

## Cashew and Blueberry Cheesecake

**Serving Yields**: 8

**Nutritional Counts**: Net Carbs: 6 g| Fat: 16 g

**Ingredients for the crust:**

- Cinnamon – 1 tsp.
- Desiccated coconut – 2 tbsp.
- Ground flaxseeds – 2 tbsp.

**Ingredients for the filling:**

- Soaked cashews – 1 cup
- Vegan-type cream cheese – 4 oz.
- Lemon juice – 1 tbsp.
- Coconut oil – 2 tbsp.
- Frozen blueberries - .5 cup
- Vanilla extract – 1 tsp.
- Liquid stevia – to your liking

**Preparation Method:**

- Mix all of the crust components and flatten using two containers.
- Combine all of the filling fixings in a blender until smooth.
- Empty the filling into the containers and chill until firm.
- Serve anytime you want a yummy treat.

## Chilled Avocado and Strawberry Bowl

**Serving Yields**: 1

**Nutritional Counts**: Net Carbs: 5 g| Fat: 10 g

**Ingredients:**

- Lime – 1 tsp.
- Peeled – pitted – avocado – 1 cup
- Pinch of salt – 1 pinch
- To Your Liking: Stevia

**Preparation Method:**

- Combine all of the goodies in a blender.
- Incorporate until smooth and place in the fridge to chill.

## Cinnamon and Pumpkin Fudge

**Serving Yields:** 25 servings

**Nutritional Counts:** Net Carbs: 2.19 g| Fat: 10.63 g

### Ingredients:

- Ground nutmeg - .25 tsp
- Ground cinnamon – 1 tsp.
- Pumpkin puree – 1 cup
- Warmed/melted coconut butter – 1.75 cups
- Coconut oil – 1 tbsp.

### Preparation Method:

- Combine the fixings (coconut butter, spices, and pumpkin). Whisk in the coconut oil.
- Spread the mixture over a foil-lined baking dish and cover with wax paper. Press out the fudge until even. Discard the paper and place in the fridge for 2 hours.
- Chop into squares and keep handy for the next sugar craving!

## Coconut Bombs

**Serving Yields**: 30

**Nutritional Counts**: Net Carbs: 1 g| Fat: 13 g

### Ingredients:

- Coconut oil - .75 cup
- Coconut milk – 1 can
- Unsweetened coconut flakes – 1 cup

- Liquid stevia – 20 drops

**Preparation Method:**

- Add the oil to a microwavable bowl. Let it cook about 20 seconds or until melted. Stir in the stevia and milk.
- Add the coconut flakes and pour into candy molds.
- Place in the freezer for one hour. Yummy!

## Coconut Cupcakes

**Serving Yields**: 7

**Nutritional Counts**: Net Carbs: 4.25 g| Fat: 30.7 g

**Ingredients:**

- Psyllium husk – 2 tbsp.
- Vanilla flavored protein powder – 4.25 oz.
- Unsweetened coconut flakes – 3 oz.
- Coconut oil – 4 tbsp.
- Unsweetened coconut milk – 6.7 oz.
- 85% cocoa – dark chocolate - .75 oz.

**Preparation Method:**

- Combine the coconut flakes, psyllium, and protein powder. Mix and blend in the coconut milk and oil. Add the mixture into cupcake forms.
- Melt the chocolate in a saucepan and drizzle the cupcakes.
- Freeze for about 30 minutes and sprinkle with the pecan halves.
- Let them firm up in the refrigerator for 2 hours.
- Cut into pieces and enjoy.
- Add a delicious low-carb frosting if desired, but count the extra carbs.

## Coconut Maple Fudge

**Serving Yields**: 18

**Nutritional Counts**: Net Carbs: 0.5 g| Fat: 9.1 g

**Ingredients:**

- Coconut oil - .5 cup
- Coconut butter - .5 cup
- Maple extract – 1 tsp.
- Shredded – unsweetened- toasted coconut - .5 cup

- Liquid stevia coconut sweet drops - .5 tsp.

**Preparation Method:**

- Add a layer of parchment paper to a baking tin.
- Melt the coconut butter and oil in a pan (low heat). Combine everything (Omit the coconut for now.).
- Sprinkle the coconut on the prepared baking sheet. Pour the batter over the mixture.
- Place in the refrigerator to firm up. Then, cut into 18 pieces and enjoy!

## Coconut and Peanut Butter Balls

**Serving Yields**: 15

**Nutritional Counts**: Net Carbs: 0.92 g| Fat: 3.19 g

**Ingredients:**

- Unsweetened cocoa powder – 3 tsp.
- Creamy peanut butter – vegan-friendly – 3 tbsp.
- Almond flour – 2 tsp.
- Powdered erythritol – 2.5 tsp.
- Unsweetened coconut flakes - .5 cup

**Preparation Method:**

- Combine the cocoa, peanut butter, erythritol, and flour.
- Place in the freezer for 1 hour.
- Using a small spoon, prepare the servings and drop into coconut flakes.

- Roll them around and reshape if needed.
- Refrigerate until firm.

## Coconut and Strawberry Bars

**Serving Yields**: 2

**Nutritional Counts**: Net Carbs: 4 g| Fat: 28 g

**Ingredients:**

- Melted coconut butter – 16 oz.
- Coconut oil – 1 tbsp.
- Chopped strawberries – 1 cup
- Coconut – dry- .25 cup
- Stevia – 1 tsp.

**Preparation Method:**

- Combine the butter, oil, and stevia to make the bowl have a 'greasy' appearance. Add the berries and garnish with the coconut.
- Place in the fridge for four hours. When chilled, cut into bars.
- Enjoy anytime you want a tasty treat.

## Dairy-Free Chocolate Silk Pie

**Serving Yields**: 8

**Nutritional Counts**: Net Carbs: 6.6 g| Fat: 41.31 g

**Ingredients:**

- Chilled coconut milk, liquid discarded – 2 cans - 13.5-oz. each
- Almond butter - .5 cup
- Vanilla extract – 1 tsp.
- Granulated erythritol - .25 cup
- Low-carb dark chocolate – 4 oz.
- Almond flour – 1 cup
- Coconut flour – 2 tbsp.
- Granulated sweetener – 2 tbsp.
- Xanthan gum – 1 tsp.
- Sea salt - .5 tsp.
- Ghee – 2 tbsp.
- Water – 1-2 tbsp.
- Slivered almonds -for the garnish – 2 tbsp.

**Preparation Method:**

- In a saucepan, heat the coconut cream, sweetener, vanilla, and almond butter until they're completely melted together.
- Take the saucepan off of the burner. Stir until the chocolate is melted and creamy smooth. Refrigerate the mixture while you prepare the crust.
- Whisk or sift the flours, sweetener, salt, and xanthan gum. Using a fork, cut in the ghee until the mixture is crumbly and beginning to resemble dough.
- Add half of the water and knead into dough. If it's looking dry, add more water, so the mixture is sticky to the touch.
- Press into a pie tin and bake at 350°F for 15 minutes or until the edges brown. Once the crust is baked, pour the chocolate filling into the pie tin and place in the freezer for at least 4 hours.
- Slice the pie and serve cold. Refrigerate any leftovers!

# Lime Avocado Popsicles

**Serving Yields**: 6

**Nutritional Counts**: Net Carbs: 3.2 g| Fat: 21.9 g

**Ingredients:**

- Erythritol - .25 cup
- Coconut milk – 1.5 cups
- Avocados - 2
- Lime juice – 2 tbsp.

**Preparation Method:**

- For a tasty treat on a hot day; simply dice the avocados into chunks and add them with the rest of the fixings to a blender. Mix until smooth.
- Pour the mixture into six popsicle molds and gently tap the container on the countertop to remove any air bubbles.
- Freeze for 7-8 hours with a stick inserted in the center of the mold.
- Run water over the mold to remove the delicious popsicle.

# Mexican Chocolate Avocado Ice Cream

**Serving Yields**: 6 (3 cups)

**Nutritional Counts**: Net Carbs: 4.16 g| Fat: 25.74 g

**Ingredients:**

- Full-fat coconut milk - 15- oz. – 1 can
- Swerve Sweetener - .33 cup
- Espresso powder - optional – 1 tsp.
- Sugar-free - chopped dark chocolate – ex. Lily's – 3 oz.
- Vanilla extract – 1 tsp.
- Medium California Avocados – 2
- Ground cinnamon – 1.5 tsp.
- Chipotle powder - .25 to .75 tsp. - depending on how spicy you like it

**Preparation Method:**

- Whisk together the sweetener and espresso powder with the milk in a pan until the sweetener has dissolved. The expresso will post the flavor of the chocolate.
- Chop the chocolate. Take the saucepan off of the burner and add the chocolate. Let it cool for about four until chocolate is melted, then whisk in the vanilla - mixing until smooth.
- Combine the cinnamon, chipotle chocolate mixture, and avocados in a blender or food processor. Puree until smooth.
- Store in the fridge for at least two hours. Transfer into an ice cream maker and churn until the consistency resembles soft serve ice cream (this takes less time than custard-based ice creams).
- Serve as soft serve or transfer to an airtight container and freeze another few hours for a firmer consistency.

## Minty Berries in A Dish

**Serving Yields**: 6

**Nutritional Counts**: Net Carbs: 8.5 g| Fat: 12 g

**Ingredients:**

- Full-fat coconut milk – 1 can
- Freshly chopped mixed berries – 4 cups
- Vanilla pod – seeds only – 1 pod
- Birch xylitol - 1 tsp.
- Fresh mint leaves - 1

**Preparation Method:**

- Mix the mint and berries in a mixing container.
- Empty the liquid from the coconut and throw it away. Place the 'hard' coconut in a bowl with the vanilla seeds.
- Using a hand mixer, mix the vanilla mixture and stevia.
- Serve the berries and cream for breakfast or a luscious dessert.

## Pecan and Blueberry Crumble

**Serving Yields**: 6

**Nutritional Counts**: Net Carbs: 15.24 g| Fat: 31.33 g

**Ingredients:**

- Chia seeds – 3 tbsp.
- Lemon juice – 1 tbsp.
- Blueberries – 14 oz.

- Stevia powder – 1.5 tsp.
- Blanched almond flour – 2 cups
- Cinnamon – 2 tbsp.
- Chopped pecans - .25 cups
- Coconut oil – 5 tbsp.

**Preparation Method:**

- Warm up the oven to 400°F.
- Prepare a cast iron skillet. Combine the berries, stevia, chia seeds, and lemon juice. Pour into the pan.
- Mix the rest of the fixings in a bowl and spread over the pan of berries.
- Add the skillet to the hot oven and bake for 30 minutes.
- Remove and portion out to six servings.

## Pumpkin Truffles

**Serving Yields**: 18

**Nutritional Counts**: Net Carbs: 1.4 g| Fat: 6.1 g

**Ingredients:**

- Pumpkin spice – 2 tsp.
- Pumpkin puree – 1.5 cups
- Softened coconut butter - .75 cup
- Vanilla extract – 1 tsp.

- Vanilla liquid stevia – 1 tsp.

**Preparation Method:**

- Prepare a baking sheet with a piece of parchment paper.
- Add all of the fixings in a blender. Once it's creamy, use a scoop and add the truffles to the baking tin.
- Place in the refrigerator until firm. Enjoy anytime!

## Raspberry Coconut Bark

**Serving Yields**: 12

**Nutritional Counts**: Net Carbs: 2.45 g| Fat: 23.56 g

**Ingredients:**

- Frozen berries - .5 cup
- Coconut oil - .5 cup
- Coconut butter - .5 cup
- Unsweetened shredded coconut - .5 cup
- Powdered swerve sweetener - .25 cup

**Preparation Method:**

- Line a baking tin with parchment paper.
- Turn the frozen berries into powder with a food processor. Set aside.
- Mix the rest of the fixings in a saucepan (low heat). Stir until melted.
- Pour ½ of the mixture into the baking pan.

- Mix the rest of the pan mixture with the powdered berries (step 2). Stir well and spoon the raspberry delight over the coconut mix and swirl with a butter knife.

- Place in the freezer until it can be easily broken into pieces (bark).

## Raspberry Truffles

**Serving Yields**: 24

**Nutritional Counts**: Net Carbs: 5.4 g| Fat: 10.8 g

**Ingredients:**
- Fresh raspberries – 1 cup
- Unsweetened cashew butter – 1 cup
- Melted coconut oil – 2 tbsp.
- Raspberry extract - .5 tsp.
- Berry liquid stevia - .5 tsp.
- 85% dark chocolate – 1 - 8 oz. portion
- Salt – 1 pinch

**Preparation Method:**
- Line a baking sheet with a sheet of baking parchment paper
- Mix all of the fixings - but omit the chocolate for now - in a food processor and pulse until smooth.
- Scoop out 24 truffles and press a raspberry in the center of each. Place on the prepared cookie sheet and freeze for 30 minutes.
- Place the chocolate in the microwave until melted (30-60 seconds).
- Dip the truffles into the melted chocolate with a skewer and place back on the baking tin. Refrigerate until ready to devour!

# Strawberry Ice Cream

**Serving Yields**: 5

**Nutritional Counts**: Net Carbs: 2 g| Fat: 13 g

**Ingredients:**

- Strawberries – 1 cup
- Water – 1 cup
- Full-fat coconut milk – 1 can
- Glucomannan powder – 1 tsp.
- Vanilla extract – 1 tsp.
- Stevia drops – as desired

**Preparation Method:**

- Using the stovetop (low heat), combine the glucomannan powder and water. Stir until it forms a gel.
- Combine all of the fixings in a blender and mix until smooth.
- Chill for one hour and transfer to an ice cream maker.
- Enjoy this dessert on a hot summer day!

## Smoothies for Almost Any Occasion

### Avocado Raspberry Smoothie

**Serving Yields:** 2

**Nutritional Counts**: Net Carbs: 12.8 g | Fat: 20 g

## Ingredients:

- Lemon juice – 3 tbsp.
- Ripened avocado - 1
- Frozen unsweetened raspberries/or your favorite - .5 cup
- Water – 1.33 cups
- Sugar equivalent – your favorite keto choice - 1 tbsp. (+) 1 tsp.

## Preparation Method:

- Combine each of the fixings in a blender until smooth.
- Pour into chilled glasses.

# Banana Bread and Blueberry Smoothie

**Serving Yields**: 2

**Nutritional Counts**: Net Carbs: 4.66 g| Fat: 23.31 g

## Ingredients:

- Chia seeds – 1 tbsp.
- Golden flaxseed meal – 3 tbsp.
- Vanilla unsweetened coconut milk – from a carton – 2 cups
- Blueberries - .25 cups
- Liquid stevia – 10 drops
- MCT oil – 2 tbsp.

- Xanthan gum - .25 tsp
- Banana extract – 1.5 tsp.

**Preparation Method:**
- Toss all of the fixings into a high-speed blender.
- Give the chia seeds and flax a few minutes to absorb the moisture.
- Blend for 1-2 minutes until everything is fully incorporated.
- Serve in a couple of chilled glasses.

## Berry Smoothie Bowl

**Serving Yields:** 1

**Nutrition Counts:** Net Carbs: 12.83 g| Fat: 54.87 g

**Ingredients:**
- Cooked beets - .25 cup
- Raspberries - .25 cup
- Protein powder – 1 scoop
- Hemp seeds – 1 tbsp.

**Preparation Method:**
- Add everything into a bowl.
- Mix well and enjoy.

## Black Currant and Strawberry Smoothie

**Serving Yields:** 1

**Nutritional Counts**: Net Carbs: 8.7 g| Fat: 17.3 g

**Ingredients:**

- Chia seeds – 2 tbsp.
- Vanilla bean - .5 of 1
- Water - .5 cup
- Fresh black currants - .5 cup
- Fresh strawberries - .25 cup
- Coconut milk - .25 cup

**Preparation Method:**

- Using a blender; add all of the fixings and blend until smooth.
- Serve in a chilled glass.

## Blueberry Sensation

**Serving Yields**: 1

**Nutritional Counts**: Net Carbs: 3 g |Fats: 21 g

**Ingredients:**

- Blueberries - .25 cup
- Coconut milk – 1 cup
- Whey protein powder – optional – 1 scoop
- Vanilla Essence – 1 tsp.

- MCT Oil – 1 tsp.

**Preparation Method:**
- For a quick burst of energy, add all of the fixings into a blender.
- Puree until it reaches the desired consistency. Add some ice if you wish.

# Like what you're reading? Want to hear this as an audio book? Click here to get this book for FREE when you join Audible!!

## https://adbl.co/2YmbdC8

### Chocolate and Mint Smoothie

**Serving Yields**: 1

**Nutritional Counts**: Net Carbs: 6.5 g | Fats: 40.3 g

**Ingredients:**
- Medium avocado - .5 of 1
- Coconut milk - .25 cup
- Unsweetened cashew/almond milk – 1 cup
- Swerve/erythritol – 2 tbsp.
- Cocoa powder – 1 tbsp.
- Several fresh mint leaves

- MCT oil – 1 tbsp.
- Ice cubes - 3
- Coconut milk/whipped cream - optional

**Preparation Method:**

- Mix all of the ingredients in your blender.
- Add ice cubes as many as you like. Add the topping if desired.
- Serve and enjoy!

## Chocolate Smoothie

**Serving Yields**: 1 Large

**Nutritional Counts**: Net Carbs: 4.4 g | Fat: 46 g

**Ingredients:**
- Chia seeds 1-2 tbsp.
- Almond or coconut butter - 1-2 tbsp.
- Egg substitute to replace 2 large eggs
- Coconut milk/heavy whipping cream - .25 cup
- Plain/chocolate whey protein - .25 cup
- Stevia extract - 3-5 drops
- Extra-virgin coconut oil - 1 tbsp.
- Unsweetened cacao powder - 1 tbsp.
- Water - .25 cup
- Ice - .5 cup
- Vanilla extract/cinnamon - .5 tsp.

**Preparation Method:**

- Combine all of the fixings into the blender.
- Pulse until frothy. Add to a chilled glass and enjoy anytime.

# Cinnamon Chocolate Smoothie

**Serving Yields**: 1

**Nutritional Counts**: Net Carbs: 4 g| Fat: 30 g

**Ingredients:**

- Ripened avocado - .5 of 1
- Coconut milk - .75 cup
- Cinnamon powder – 1 tsp.
- Vanilla extract - .25 tsp.
- Unsweetened cocoa powder – 2 tsp.
- Stevia – as desired
- Optional: Coconut oil – 1 tsp. or MCT oil - .5 tsp.
- Ice – 1 cup

**Preparation Method:**

- Mix all of the fixings in a blender. Lastly, empty the ice.
- Blend on the high setting for 30 seconds until thickened or until thickened.

# Cinnamon Roll Smoothie

**Serving Yields**: 1

**Nutritional Counts**: Net Carbs: 0.6 g |Fats: 3.25 g

## Ingredients:

- Vanilla protein powder – 2 tbsp.
- Flax meal – 1 tsp.
- Almond milk – 1 cup
- Vanilla extract - .25 tsp.
- Sweetener – 4 tsp.
- Cinnamon - .5 tsp.
- Ice – 1 cup

## Preparation Method:

- Mix all of the fixings in a blender. Lastly, empty the ice.
- Blend on the high setting for 30 seconds until thickened or until thickened.

# Easter Time Smoothie

**Serving Yields**: 1
**Nutritional Counts**: Net Carbs: 10.8 g| Fat: 23.3 g

## Ingredients:

- Cantaloupe or honeydew - 1 small wedge or 1.8 oz. total
- Coconut milk/full-fat cream - .25 cup
- Avocado – 1.8 oz. - average sized
- Psyllium/chia seeds – 1 tbsp.
- Kiwifruit/berries - .25 cup
- Plain or vanilla whey protein - .25 cup

- Liquid stevia extract – 2-6 drops
- Water - .5 cup
- Ice chunks if desired – 2-3

**Preparation Method:**

- Cut the avocado in half and scoop out the insides; add it to a blender.
- Toss in the kiwi, peeled melon, and the remainder of the goodies.
- Blend well and enjoy!

## Green Choco Smoothies

**Serving Yields**: 2

**Nutritional Counts**: Net Carbs: 5.8 g| Fat: 16.3 g

**Ingredients:**

- Coconut cream – 1 cup
- Frozen berries - .5 cup
- Cocoa powder - .25 cup
- Granulated sweetener – 1 tbsp.

**Preparation Method:**

- Use a high-speed blender to combine all of the fixings.
- Blend until you have reached the desired consistency.
- Serve in a couple of chilled glasses.

## Maca Almond Smoothie

**Serving Yields**: 1

**Nutritional Counts**: Net Carbs: 6.2 g| Fat: 43.8 g

### Ingredients:

- Unsweetened almond milk - .75 cup
- Coconut milk - .25 cup
- Unsweetened almond butter – 1 tbsp.
- Collagen powder – 1 tbsp.
- Extra-Virgin olive oil – 1 tbsp.
- Maca powder – 2 tsp.

### Preparation Method:

- Combine all of the fixings in a blender.
- Mix well until smooth and serve in a chilled mug.

## Minty Avocado and Spinach Smoothie

**Serving Yields**: 1

**Nutritional Counts**: Net Carbs: 3.6 g| Fat: 13.3 g

### Ingredients:

- Fresh spinach – 1 cup
- Unsweetened almond milk - .5 cup
- Avocado - .5 of 1
- Whey protein powder – 1 scoop
- Stevia – 10 drops
- Peppermint extract - .25 tsp.
- Ice – 1 cup

**Preparation Method:**

- Combine the milk, spinach, avocado, stevia, whey powder, extract, and ice in a blender.
- Mix well until creamy, just the way you like it!

## Pumpkin and Avocado Smoothie

**Serving Yields**: 1

**Nutritional Counts**: Net Carbs: 11.3 g| Fat: 69.8 g

**Ingredients:**

- Pumpkin puree – 3 tbsp.
- Coconut milk - full-fat - .75 cup
- MCT oil – 1 tbsp.
- Freshly chopped avocado - .5 of 1
- Pumpkin spice - .5 tsp.
- Vanilla – alcohol-free – 1 tsp.

**Preparation Method:**

- Add all of the fixings to a blender.
- Mix well until creamy smooth.
- *Special Tip*: Not only will you enjoy the vibrant color; the pumpkin converts any ingested beta-carotene into vitamin A. This is a plus to help reduce the risk of some cancers, heart disease, and asthma.

## Spinach and Cucumber Smoothie

**Serving Yields**: 1

**Nutritional Counts**: Net Carbs: 2.91 g| Fat: 32.34 g

**Ingredients:**

- Cucumber – 2.5 oz.
- Spinach –2 handfuls.
- Coconut milk – from a carton – 1 cup
- Cubes of ice – 7 Large
- Liquid stevia – 12 drops
- MCT Oil – 1-2 tbsp.
- Xanthan gum - .25 tsp.

**Preparation Method:**

- Peel and cube the cucumber. Combine all of the fixings in a high-speed blender (ex. Ninja).
- Blend for 1-2 minutes until it's creamy like you like it.
- Pour into a chilled glass and enjoy the healthy drink anytime!

# Cold Beverages

## Green Coffee Shake

**Serving Yields**: 4

**Nutritional Counts**: Net Carbs: 4.4 g| Fat: 24.9 g

**Ingredients:**

- Full-fat coconut milk - 1 can - 13.5 fl. oz.
- Chilled brewed coffee (decaf or regular – 1.5 cup
- Unsweetened almond butter – 2 tbsp.
- Genuine Health vegan greens - vanilla-flavored – 1 tbsp.
- For Serving: Ice cubes - 8

**Preparation Method:**

- Combine all of the fixings except for the ice in the blender jug.
- Pulse until smooth or about 10 seconds.
- Portion into your chosen glasses and add the ice cubes.
- Serve and smile!

## Iced Blended Coffee

**Serving Yields**: 1

**Nutritional Counts**: Net Carbs: 64.7 g| Fat: 99.3 g

**Ingredients:**

- Hemp hearts – 2 tbsp. or 1 tbsp. almond butter
- Brewed coffee/favorite tea – 1.75 cups
- Cacao butter -10 g. – 4-5 wafers
- Alcohol-free stevia – 4 drops
- Coconut- 1 tbsp. or MCT oil
- Ground cinnamon - .25 tsp.
- Ground vanilla bean - .25 tsp
- Cubes of ice – 4-6

**Ingredients for the topping:**

- Cacao nibs – 1 tsp.
- Coconut whipped cream - .25 cup

**Preparation Method:**

- Measure out all of the fixings and add to a blender; mix until creamy smooth.
- Toss in the ice and continue until it's the way you like it.
- Serve with the chosen toppings.

## McKeto Strawberry Milkshake

**Serving Yields**: 1

**Nutritional Counts:** Net Carbs: 2.42 g| Fat: 38.85

**Ingredients:**

- Heavy cream - .25 cup

- Coconut milk – from a carton - .75 cup
- Sugar-free Strawberry Torani Syrup – 2 tbsp.
- Xanthan gum - .25 tsp.
- MCT oil – 1 tbsp.
- Cubes of ice - 7

**Preparation Method:**

- Combine all of the fixings in a blender. (such as Ninja).
- Combine for 1-2 minutes until it's like you enjoy it.
- Serve in a chilled glass.

## Hot Beverages

### Coconut – Coffee Mug

**Serving Yields**: 1

**Nutritional Counts**: Net Carbs: 2 g| Fat: 27 g

**Ingredients:**

- Coconut oil – 1 tbsp.
- Ground flaxseeds – 2 tbsp.
- Coconut flakes – unsweetened – 2 tbsp.
- Liquid sweetener – as desired
- Unsweetened black coffee - .5 cup

**Preparation Method:**

- Combine the flaxseeds, coconut oil, and coconut flakes in a mug.
- Pour in the prepared coffee. Add the sweetener of choice and enjoy.

## Creamy Hot Cocoa in the Crockpot

**Serving Yields**: 4

**Nutritional Counts**: Net Carbs: 3 g| Fat: 5 g

**Ingredients:**
- Unsweetened almond milk – 3 cups
- Salt - .25 tsp.
- Stevia – 8-10 packets
- Vanilla – 1 tsp.
- Half and Half - .25 cup
- Cocoa powder – unsweetened - .25 cup (+) 2 tbsp.

**Preparation Method:**
- Combine all of the fixings in the crockpot.
- Set the timer for two hours using the low setting (covered).
- Stir occasionally. Serve in a warm mug and enjoy!

## Energizing Latte

**Serving Yields**: 1

**Nutritional Counts**: Net Carbs: -0- g| Fat: 25.8 g

**Ingredients:**

- Stevia – 1 drop
- Brewed coffee – 8 oz.
- Cacao butter - 1 tbsp.
- Hemp hearts - 1 tbsp.
- MCT oil - 1 tbsp.
- Grass-fed collagen - 1 tbsp.

**Preparation Method:**

- First, brew the coffee and combine all of the fixings in a blender (omit the collagen).
- Mix for 1 minute and add the collagen (the last 10 sec.).
- Enjoy before you start your hectic day.

# A Final Word

You now have a ton of recipes to choose from as a vegan. Before you begin, it is advisable to visit your doctor. If you are attempting to lose weight using the ketogenic diet techniques, you need to be aware of some possible medications that can contribute to weight gain. Do you take any of these?

- Oral contraceptives
- Anti-Depressants
- Epilepsy drugs
- Blood pressure medications
- Allergy medicines
- Antibiotics

As you begin your dieting using your keto lifestyle changes, you will notice some obvious differences. Here are some examples:

## Keto Flu

The diet can make you a bit confused, irritable, nauseous, cause you to have diarrhea or constipation, muscle cramping, bloated, and lethargic. You may also suffer from a lingering headache. Sugar cravings and heart palpations may also be present. Just like the traditional flu, the keto flu may have a total run of 24-72-hours. Several days into the plan should remedy these issues. If not, just add 1/2 teaspoon of salt to a glass of water. Drink it to help ease the side effects. It might be necessary to do this once a day for about the first week.

Note: It could take about 15-20 minutes before it helps.

## Intense urine odor

The color change is due to your body adjusting and entering ketosis.

## Adjustments in the digestive system

As your body is challenged by additional fiber and other foods, you may experience bouts of constipation or diarrhea. Water also helps with dehydration but may also cause intestinal issues. Try reducing new foods until the transitional phase of ketosis is concluded; it should clear up with time. You may also be lacking beneficial bacteria. Try consuming fermented foods to increase your probiotics and aid digestion. You can also benefit from Vitamin B, omega-3 fatty acids, and beneficial enzymes. Take a dose of Milk of Magnesia if other suggestions don't work for you.

### Heart palpitations

It is possible you will have heart palpitations as a result of insufficient intake of salt or dehydration. Adjust your menu plan with a few more carbs to see if they subside. If you don't begin to feel better soon, you should seek emergency care.

### Changes in sleeping pattern

If you have been asleep for over eight hours; that good night of sleep will throw your body into ketosis. If you are new to the low-carb and high-fat diet plan, it will take time to achieve optimal fat-burning status. Your body has depended on bringing in carbs and glucose; it will not readily give up carbs and start to crave saturated fats. Insomnia is a normal side effect.

Vitamin supplements can sometimes remedy the problem that can be caused by a lowered insulin and serotonin level. For a quick fix, try one-half of a tablespoon of fruit spread and a square of chocolate. It really does work! However, you still need to count the carbs (if any) of your homemade remedy.

Don't eat dinner when it's close to bedtime. You should consume the last meal of the day approximately two to three hours before it's time to retire for the day. If you're prone to Gastroesophageal Reflux Disease or GERD, eating before bed is also a sure-fire way of making the matter worse, even a snack will cause issues. Try half of an egg, cherry tomatoes, or a few almonds if you cannot make it to the next meal.

### Insomnia

If you have problems sleeping a full eight hours, then you are like about 75% of Americans. According to the Centers for Disease Control and Prevention (CDC), that equals to about one out of three people who could have issues with type 2 diabetes, cardiovascular disease, obesity, or high blood pressure/hypertension because of the lack of sleep.

Therefore, the less sleep you get, the harder it is to drop those extra pounds. According to another study, individuals who slept just four hours experienced a 24% jump in calorie intake, increased hunger drive, decreased leptin levels (the appetite control hormone), and increased ghrelin levels (the appetite hormone that triggers hunger).

You tend to snack more and add up those calories quickly without the right amount of restful sleep. These are a few of the elements that could be causing your sleepless nights:

- Substance or alcohol abuse
- Certain illnesses
- Depression, anxiety, and stress
- Hormonal conditions and changes
- Sleep apnea
- Certain medications
- Stimulants, including too much caffeine

If you have insomnia and cannot sleep, have a serving of **Spiced Hot Toddy** for zero carbs; it only takes about ten minutes.

### Spiced Hot Toddy

**Nutrition Facts**: 110 Calories

> Note: You have -0- g Protein, Total Fats, and Net Carbs

**What You Need**:

- Bourbon – 1.5 oz.
- Boiling water – 2 oz.
- Fresh lemon juice - .25 of 1
- Whole cloves – 2

- Sweetener of choice – to taste
- Cinnamon stick – 1
- Garnish with a dash of ground nutmeg

**How to Prepare:**
- Combine all of the liquid components in a small pot on the stovetop.
- Lower the heat and add the spices and cinnamon stick. Simmer for about 3 minutes. Sprinkle with a dusting of nutmeg.
- When ready, just pour into a mug to kick your worst cold (or anything else).
- You can make multiple servings in a crockpot if you want to serve the crowd. Just keep the lid on the cooker.
- Note: Just remember, this is not an open invitation to drink alcohol; it is just one option to consider.

**Risks for those with diabetes**

If you are diabetic and want to begin a ketogenic diet plan, there are a few things you need to keep in mind. The keto diet has proven benefits for individuals who have type 2 diabetes, but you should be a bit more cautious if you have type 1 diabetes. There is not as much research at this time on other forms of diabetes.

Keep in mind that it's the quality, not the quantity, of the carbs you consume since you do not want to slice them from your diet plan entirely. Have a talk with your doctor to help you make a healthy choice for your needs.

Don't cut out the carbs too quickly. According to Prevention, it isn't wise to dramatically cut carbs from your diet, especially if you are taking insulin or oral diabetes medications. This could result in low blood glucose (hypoglycemia). You want to lower the carb intake gradually.

Don't consume too many carbs either. You need to be sure you follow a strict carb count guideline since you don't realize how many points each food has and how quickly they add up. In addition to other side effects, you will also have bouts of constipation, keto flu, or possible dehydration. However, these are just small bumps in the road for most individuals.

Be aware of diabetic ketoacidosis. According to Mayo Clinic, when diabetics produce high levels of ketones, it can potentially become a severe complication. This triggers when your body does not receive an appropriate amount of insulin which converts the sugar into energy. Therefore, if it goes into "starvation mode," it will break down the fuel at an alarmingly fast rate. Don't take the chance, stay in touch with your doctor for the best results using the ketogenic way of living.

## Keep Your Final Goals in Mind While on the Keto Journey

It is a long trip to keep and maintain ketosis. This segment is a reminder of the essential elements for you to have a smooth transition to ketosis and beyond.

### Expect plateaus with your weight loss plan

If you have ever dieted before, you already know you will reach spans of time where your weight loss will reach a level out. That's merely a segment of weight loss that can't be moderated. All you need to do is remain consistent; the weight loss will return.

### Practice mindful eating

It is vital to take a few extra moments to enjoy the flavors and textures of your food. The ketogenic diet will provide all of the nourishment to remain successful dieting. Enjoy your time with the conversation of a friend or family member. Drink your water and sip your tea or coffee. Feel satisfied and enjoy the moment; stop rushing around at dinner time.

### Limit psychological and physical stress during evening hours

It is essential for you to recharge and take the evening hours to relax to improve your sleep hygiene. Try to leave work – at work; deal with the issues in the morning. If you are going through a tough time or working long hours, you tend to forget items you may "munch" on as you are working. Make it a point to write down everything you eat.

Working long hours can be beneficial for knocking off those pounds. However, it can also cause you to be restless and can lead to post-workout insomnia if you have done strenuous physical activities on your evenings off. No matter what the case, slow down for at least an hour or more before attempting to retire for the evening.

### Limit your screen time and dim the lights

Your production of melatonin has a negative impact if the blue screen lights are left on your computer, tablets, or cell phone. Shut it all down about an hour before bedtime. You might not be able to shut the phone down completely, but use an app that will lower the lighting. The thought of missing a call can keep your mind wired at alert which will make sleep more difficult. In short, limit your exposure to the blue lights.

### Reassess and adjust your goals as needed

After you have adjusted your body to the ketogenic dieting plan, you can start using an intermittent fasting method if you choose to take that route. Be willing to change your goals as you make progress. By starting small, you leave the door open so you can make more significant challenges as you proceed through the plan.

### Always remain honest with yourself

Even though the ketogenic foods will provide you with essential vitamins and nutrients without a lot of junk foods, it doesn't necessarily mean that it is automatically the right option for your needs.

Think about how disciplined you are, what your relationship with food is like, and how healthy you are in general. It is a lot easier to be realistic about your chance of success and decide to look elsewhere before you get started in earnest than after struggling with and failing after a week or more of serious effort. With Keto, you will be satisfied and less likely to fail versus other dieting methods. You have many choices to succeed in your weight loss regimen.

### Take a break

When starting out, it is essential to understand that the transition period can be somewhat tricky, and it will be worse for some. As such, it is a good idea to choose a time to start the transition that is relatively free from stress or otherwise hectic plans. You are likely going to have a hard time making the change. Anything else on your plate is probably going to take a hit. "Forewarned is forearmed," however, and planning for the development will make it easier to manage.

### Reward yourself

Especially when you are first starting out, it is important to reward a successful week on your new way of eating with some type of splurge. As long as you don't let it get out of hand, there is no harm in having an extra decadent dessert; just make sure it remains in the keto carb levels. Better yet, go on a new adventure with the family.

## More about those plateaus

Okay, you have made it this far, and you realize there will be bumps in the road during your time headed toward ketosis. These are a few that others have made so you can dodge them. This is always a good review time!

### Plateau 1: Not tracking your carbs properly

As you enter into ketosis, your hunger generation is generally improved. Since ketogenic foods can be calorically-dense, you need to be sure that you are tracking and weighing all of your food. That's the only way you will maintain a deficit.

### Plateau 2: Not eating the right veggie and fruit choices

It's pretty simple to avoid this issue with a side of broccoli or cauliflower. You can also have a healthy side salad here or some of the delicious fruits provided in your previous chapters.

### Plateau 3: Not having an actual deficit

Once you have lost an adequate amount of weight, it might be essential to reassess your macros. Since you weigh much less, you will also need to lower your food consumption.

### Plateau 4: Snacking mindlessly

Make sure you are genuinely hungry before you decide to splurge. Have a large glass of water. You have to be mindful since snacking can be caused by negative emotions or just plain boredom. Food is for fuel to run your body. Therefore, eating when you aren't hungry might distort your body's natural cues. After all, hunger is a part of the weight loss equation. Your body likes the balance and wants to hold onto its current weight. That is why, on some days, you may be hungrier than others. Power through those weak moments or enjoy a healthy snack.

### Plateau 5: Watch out for hidden carbs

Remember the ideal carb consumption is at or below 20-25 net carbs while using the keto plan – especially when you begin your diet plan. Be sure you are tracking the carbs and not eating too many foods that might have carbohydrates lurking. As an example, tofu can have different carbs depending on the brand. Always check your labels when shopping for your keto needs.

# Benefits of Ketogenic Diet as a Vegan

### Seizure reduction for epilepsy patients
Reductions in seizures have occurred in children who have successfully used the ketogenic diet. The therapeutic keto diet used for epilepsy often restricts the carbs to fewer than 15 grams of carbs daily to further drive up the ketone levels. Don't try to reach these levels unless you have the supervision of a medical professional.

### Accelerated fat loss for overweight and obese individuals
Many people exceed what is considered healthy figures when it comes to weight. It is imperative to use the keto diet plan to get started on the right path for weight loss.

### Prediabetes and diabetes improvements
With the excess fat removed using the keto plan, you will also have noted improvement of pre-diabetes, type-2 diabetes, and metabolic syndrome.

### Joint pain and stiffness is significantly improved
Grain-based foods are abolished from your diet using the keto plan. It's believed the grains can be one of the biggest causes of pain or chronic illness.

### Improved thinking skills
You might become confused as you consume high-fat foods since your brain is approximately 60% fat by weight. It can maintain itself and work at full capacity using ketosis.

### Cancer patient relief
Several types of cancer and slow tumor growths are being treated by using the keto diet technique.

### A slowed process of those with Alzheimer's disease
The disease's progression can be delayed and the symptoms reduced with the keto plan.

### Lower blood pressures
It is wise to speak with your doctor about lowering your medications while on the plan. If you begin to feel dizzy, this is an indication that the lack of carbs is working.

### Cholesterol profile improvement
An arterial buildup is typically associated with the triglyceride and cholesterol levels, which have been proven to improve with the keto diet plan.

**Repaired gum disease and tooth decay issues**
The pH balance in your mouth is influenced by sugar intake. The plan should help your gum issues subside after about three months.

# Conclusion

I hope each segment of the Vegan Keto Cookbook was informative and able to provide you with all the tools you need to achieve whatever your goals may be. If you are searching for a well-rounded diet for your child, these tips could be useful for training the way of a vegan diet:

- Let the children help.
- Start the process with foods the child already likes.
- Provide a packed lunch, so you would know your child has the right types of foods.
- Mix up the menu and keep it interesting.
- Plan meals in advance.

Keep it simple for children; try some of these great finger foods:

- Pear slices
- Apple slices
- Banana
- Avocado
- Sweet potato cubes and slices
- Carrot sticks and rounds

Keep track of which foods are best liked by your child. Always keep a watch while you provide the crunchy snacks. Some of these foods will require adult supervision. As with any diet, you may have side effects. The ketogenic plan offers several ways to remedy the issues.

The next step is to decide which deliciously healthy meal you want to try first and prepare a list of each of the ingredients you need. It is also advisable to make a list of staples which will be used with many of the vegan type recipes. You can use the information provided within to prepare tasty dishes that your family and friends will rave about for quite some time. You have the total fats and net carbs calculated by Keto standards, so have fun!

Finally, if you found *"The Vegan Keto Cookbook: Over 190 High-Fat Low-Carb Plant-Based Recipes to Shed and Heal You from the Inside Out"* useful in any way, a review on Amazon is always appreciated!

# Index for the Recipes

## Chapter 1: Morning and Brunch Specialties

- *Bulletproof Coffee* ............................................................................... *18*
- *Bulletproof Tea* ................................................................................... *20*

**Pancake and Waffle Time** ........................................................................ **21**

- *Cinnamon Roll Pancakes* ................................................................... *21*
- *Coconut Pancakes* .............................................................................. *23*
- *Crispy Flaxseed Waffles* ..................................................................... *24*
- *Flaxseed Pancakes* .............................................................................. *26*
- *Scallion Pancakes* ............................................................................... *27*

**Other Delicious Choices** ........................................................................ **28**

- *Almonds and Chips Breakfast Cereal* ............................................... *28*
- *Avocado – Carrot and Tahini Breakfast Bowl* ................................. *29*
- *Bagel Thins for Breakfast* .................................................................. *30*
- *Berry and Nut Cereal* ......................................................................... *32*
- *Blueberry Breakfast Cake – Flourless and Gluten-Free* ................. *33*
- *Bran Muffins – Gluten-Free* ............................................................. *35*
- *Breakfast Quiche* ................................................................................ *37*
- *Cinnamon Roll Muffins* ..................................................................... *38*
- *Macadamia Breakfast Bars* ................................................................ *40*
- *Maple Walnut Breakfast Cereal* ........................................................ *41*
- *Minty Eggplant Hash Browns* ........................................................... *42*
- *Muesli in the Raw* ............................................................................... *43*
- *Peanut Butter Breakfast Cereal* ........................................................ *44*

- *Psyllium Breakfast Mix* .................................................................. 45
- *Pumpkin Pie Breakfast Cereal* ....................................................... 46
- *Scrambled Tofu* ............................................................................. 47
- *Seed and Nut-Packed Bread* .......................................................... 48
- *Vanilla and Turmeric Breakfast Cereal* ......................................... 50

**Oatmeal and Porridge Favorites** ............................................................. 51
- *Berries and Hemp Seeds* ................................................................ 51
- *Blueberry Porridge* ........................................................................ 52
- *Fudge Oatmeal* .............................................................................. 54

**Overnight Oat Options** ........................................................................... 55
- *Alternative #1: Vanilla Oats: The Base* ......................................... 55
- *Alternative #2: Pumpkin Spice Latte Overnight Oats* .................. 56
- *Alternative #3: Fudge Overnight Oats* .......................................... 57

**Porridge Options** ..................................................................................... 58
- *Delicious Plain Porridge*         58
- *Porridge with Cinnamon and Hemp Hearts*         59

## Chapter 2: Delicious Meals and Salads

**Meals** ........................................................................................................ 60
- *Asparagus and Mushrooms with Cauliflower Risotto* .................. 60
- *Asparagus and Tofu Stir Fry* ......................................................... 63
- *Broccoli Noodles and Tofu* ............................................................ 64
- *Cauliflower Tabbouleh* .................................................................. 66
- *Collard Green Wraps* ..................................................................... 67
- *Crispy Tofu and Cauliflower Rice* .................................................. 68
- *Eggplant Lasagna* .......................................................................... 70

- *Falafel with Tahini Sauce* .................................................................. *72*
- *French Style Ratatouille* ..................................................................... *74*
- *Green Panini* ........................................................................................ *76*
- *Sesame Tofu and Eggplant* ................................................................ *77*

**Salads** ............................................................................................................ **79**

- *Arugula and Blueberry Salad* ............................................................ *79*
- *Asian Zucchini Salad* .......................................................................... *80*
- *Asparagus and Artichoke Salad* ........................................................ *81*
- *Avocado and Greens Salad* ................................................................ *82*
- *Avocado Papaya Salad* ....................................................................... *83*
- *Bell Pepper and Asparagus Salad* ..................................................... *84*
- *Caesar Vegan Salad* ............................................................................ *85*
- *Courgette Salad and Herbed Vinaigrette* ........................................ *86*
- *Eggplant Salad* ..................................................................................... *87*
- *Kale Salad and Blueberry Dressing* .................................................. *88*
- *Lemony Brussel Sprout Salad* ............................................................ *90*
- *Pear and Dates with Special Cider Dressing* .................................. *91*
- *Pecan Cauliflower Salad* .................................................................... *92*
- *Simple Green Salad with Lemon Vinaigrette* ................................. *93*
- *Sun-Dried Tomato Salad and Cider Dressing* ................................ *95*
- *Thai Peanut Zucchini Noodle Salad* ................................................ *96*

## Chapter 3: Healthy Soups – Stews and Chowder

- *Beetroot Ginger Soup* ......................................................................... *98*
- *Broccoli and Cauliflower Soup* ........................................................ *100*
- *Cabbage and Beet Soup* .................................................................... *101*

- *Chili – Vegan Style* ........................................................................... 102
- *Chilled Minty Avocado Soup* ......................................................... 103
- *Creamy Avocado Soup* .................................................................. 104
- *Creamy Red Gazpacho Soup* ......................................................... 105
- *Creamy Tomato Soup* .................................................................... 107
- *Ginger Cauliflower Stew* ................................................................ 109
- *Mushroom Soup* ............................................................................. 110
- *Red Onion Soup* ............................................................................. 112
- *Spanish Soup* .................................................................................. 113
- *Spinach and Turnip Soup* ............................................................... 114
- *Superfood Keto Soup* ..................................................................... 115
- *Thai Pumpkin Soup* ........................................................................ 117
- *Turmeric Cabbage Soup* ................................................................. 119
- *Zucchini Basil Soup* ........................................................................ 120

## Chapter 4: Vegan Creams - Sauces and Dips

- *Avocado Mayo* ................................................................................. 121
- *Barbecue Sauce* ............................................................................... 122
- *Coconut Whipped Cream* ............................................................... 123
- *Eggplant Bruschetta* ....................................................................... 124
- *Guacamole* ...................................................................................... 125
- *Hummus and Avocado* ................................................................... 126
- *Ketchup* ........................................................................................... 127
- *Lemon and Jalapeno Cream Sauce* ................................................ 128
- *Mayo – Vegan Style* ........................................................................ 129
- *Nutella Spread* ................................................................................ 130

- *Peanut Sauce* ............................................................................................ *131*
- *Portobello Mushroom Bruschetta* ......................................................... *132*
- *Slow-Cooked Summer Bruschetta* ........................................................ *133*
- *Spinach Avocado Dip* ............................................................................ *134*
- *Tahini and Cilantro Sauce* .................................................................... *136*
- *Tofu or Seitan Marinades* ..................................................................... *137*
- *Vegan Sour Cream* ................................................................................ *140*
- *Veggie Salsa* ........................................................................................... *141*

## Chapter 5: Appetizers – Sides and Snacks

**Sides**........................................................................................................**142**

- *Basil Zoodles and Olives* ....................................................................... *142*
- *Beetroot and Pesto Noodles* .................................................................. *143*
- *Brussels Sprouts and Cashew Dip* ........................................................ *144*
- *Cabbage Slaw* ........................................................................................ *145*

*100. Carrot and Zucchini Noodles in Thai Sauce* ..................................... *146*

*101. Cauliflower and Artichoke Couscous* ................................................. *147*

*102. Cauliflower Bites with Ranch Dip* ...................................................... *148*

*103. Cherry Tomatoes and Zucchini Pasta* ............................................... *149*

*104. Chili and Coconut Cauliflower Rice* .................................................. *150*

*105. Coconut Cauliflower Rice* ................................................................... *151*

*106. Creamy Curry Low-Carb Noodle Bowl* ............................................. *152*

*107. Edamame Kelp Noodles* ..................................................................... *154*

*108. Garlicky Mushrooms* ........................................................................... *155*

*109. Grilled Eggplant and Zucchini* ........................................................... *156*

*110. Indian Curried Cauliflower* ................................................................. *157*

111. Kelp Noodles with Peanut Butter Sauce ............................................. 158

112. Lime and Chili Carrot Noodles ............................................................... 159

113. Mediterranean Spaghetti Squash ........................................................ 160

114. Mushroom, Broccoli, and Squash Noodles ....................................... 161

115. Nutty Pesto Zucchini ................................................................................. 162

116. Pesto Kelp Noodles ................................................................................... 163

117. Roasted Beetroot Noodles ..................................................................... 164

118. Roasted Broccoli ........................................................................................ 165

119. Roasted Green Cabbage ........................................................................ 166

120. Roasted Kale and Squash ...................................................................... 167

121. Spaghetti Squash ...................................................................................... 168

122. Sriracha Grilled Asparagus ................................................................... 169

123. Teriyaki Grilled Eggplant ...................................................................... 170

124. Tofu Pizza Sticks ........................................................................................ 171

125. Turnip Fries ................................................................................................. 172

126. Turnip and Courgette Hash Browns .................................................. 173

127. Zucchini Noodles and Avocado Sauce ............................................. 174

**Snack Time Treats** ......................................................................................... **175**

128. Carrot Cake Bites ...................................................................................... 175

129. Chocolate Granola .................................................................................... 176

130. Chocolate Protein Bars ........................................................................... 177

131. Cinnamon Granola ................................................................................... 178

132. Coconut and Peanut Butter Balls ....................................................... 179

133. Fudge Balls .................................................................................................. 180

134. Loaded Nut-Packed Coconut Granola ............................................. 181

135. Mushroom Chips ...................................................................................... 182

136. Pecan and Maple Fat Bars ..................................................................... 183

*137. Peanut Butter Fat Bombs* ............................................................... *184*

*138. Peanut Tofu Wrap* ....................................................................... *185*

*139. Roasted Radish Chips* ................................................................. *186*

*140. Sweet Potato Toast* ..................................................................... *187*

*141. Zucchini Chips* ............................................................................. *188*

## Chapter 6: Desserts – Smoothies and Beverages

**Pudding Specialties** ................................................................... **189**

*142. Avocado and Chocolate Pudding* ............................................... *189*

*143. Chia Chocolate Pudding* ............................................................ *191*

*144. Chia Raspberry Pudding* ........................................................... *192*

*145. Chia Strawberry Pudding* .......................................................... *193*

*146. Coconut Chia and Turmeric Pudding* ...................................... *194*

*147. Pumpkin and Peanut Butter Pudding* ..................................... *195*

**Other Delicious Desserts** .......................................................... **196**

*148. Avocado Chocolate Mousse* ...................................................... *196*

*149. Banana Bread* ............................................................................. *197*

*150. Cashew and Blueberry Cheesecake* ........................................ *198*

*151. Chilled Avocado and Strawberry Bowl* .................................. *199*

*152. Cinnamon and Pumpkin Fudge* ............................................... *200*

*153. Coconut Bombs* .......................................................................... *201*

*154. Coconut Cupcakes* ..................................................................... *202*

*155. Coconut Maple Fudge* ............................................................... *204*

*156. Coconut and Peanut Butter Balls* ............................................ *205*

*157. Coconut and Strawberry Bars* .................................................. *206*

*158. Dairy-Free Chocolate Silk Pie* ................................................... *207*

- 159. Lime Avocado Popsicles ... 209
- 160. Mexican Chocolate Avocado Ice Cream ... 210
- 161. Minty Berries in A Dish ... 211
- 162. Pecan and Blueberry Crumble ... 212
- 163. Pumpkin Truffles ... 213
- 164. Raspberry Coconut Bark ... 214
- 165. Raspberry Truffles ... 215
- 166. Strawberry Ice Cream ... 216

**Smoothies for Almost Any Occasion ... 217**

- 167. Avocado Raspberry Smoothie ... 217
- 168. Banana Bread and Blueberry Smoothie ... 218
- 169. Berry Smoothie Bowl ... 219
- 170. Black Currant and Strawberry Smoothie ... 220
- 171. Blueberry Sensation ... 221
- 172. Chocolate and Mint Smoothie ... 222
- 173. Chocolate Smoothie ... 223
- 174. Cinnamon Chocolate Smoothie ... 224
- 175. Cinnamon Roll Smoothie ... 225
- 176. Easter Time Smoothie ... 226
- 177. Green Choco Smoothies ... 227
- 178. Maca Almond Smoothie ... 228
- 179. Minty Avocado and Spinach Smoothie ... 229
- 180. Pumpkin and Avocado Smoothie ... 230
- 181. Spinach and Cucumber Smoothie ... 231

**Cold Beverages ... 232**

- 182. Green Coffee Shake ... 232
- 183. Iced Blended Coffee ... 233

*184. McKeto Strawberry Milkshake* ............................................................. *234*

## Hot Beverages ........................................................................................ **235**

*185. Coconut – Coffee Mug* ......................................................................... *235*

*186. Creamy Hot Cocoa in the Crockpot* ..................................................... *236*

*187. Energizing Latte* .................................................................................. *237*

# Keto Diet For Beginners

*Achieve Rapid Weight Loss and Burn Fat Forever in Just 21 Days with the Ketogenic Diet - Lose Up to 21 Pounds in 3 Weeks*

Tyler MacDonald

**Copyright 2019 by Tyler MacDonald - All rights reserved.**

This Book is provided with the sole purpose of providing relevant information on a specific topic for which every reasonable effort has been made to ensure that it is both accurate and reasonable. Nevertheless, by purchasing this Book, you consent to the fact that the author, as well as the publisher, are in no way experts on the topics contained herein, regardless of any claims as such that may be made within. As such, any suggestions or recommendations that are made within are done so purely for entertainment value. It is recommended that you always consult a professional prior to undertaking any of the advice or techniques discussed within.

This is a legally binding declaration that is considered both valid and fair by both the Committee of Publishers Association and the American Bar Association and should be considered as legally binding within the United States.

The reproduction, transmission, and duplication of any of the content found herein, including any specific or extended information will be done as an illegal act regardless of the end form the information ultimately takes. This includes copied versions of the work both physical, digital and audio unless express consent of the Publisher is provided beforehand. Any additional rights reserved.

Furthermore, the information that can be found within the pages described forthwith shall be considered both accurate and truthful when it comes to the recounting of facts. As such, any use, correct or incorrect, of the provided information will render the Publisher free of responsibility as to the actions taken outside of their direct purview. Regardless, there are zero scenarios where the original author or the Publisher can be deemed liable in any fashion for any damages or hardships that may result from any of the information discussed herein.

Additionally, the information in the following pages is intended only for informational purposes and should thus be thought of as universal. As befitting its nature, it is presented without assurance regarding its prolonged validity or interim quality. Trademarks that are mentioned are done without written consent and can in no way be considered an endorsement from the trademark holder.

# Introduction

Using this book as a guide will help you to easily make a lifestyle change that millions of others have already made. You will be amazed at how great you look and feel by eating foods that are delicious, healthy, and natural. You will discover its physical and mental benefits, and you will unlock a constant supply of energy.

In order to be successful with the keto diet, you will have to understand the basics of your body and how dieting works.

Many people have tried South Beach, Mediterranean, low-fat, low-calorie, Paleo, Weight Watchers, and so on. Most of them will require you to starve yourself, eat boring foods, strictly keep track of numbers, or go through a bunch of phases. The problem with the vast majority of diets is that they aren't always nutritionally sound, and they are definitely not all that satisfying. This makes them unsustainable and possibly unsafe. They aren't conducive for a happy lifestyle.

The most successful diets tend to be those who reduce your consumption of carb-rich foods. Studies have found that those who reduce their carb intake and don't change their calorie intake will lose more weight than those who follow a low-fat diet and reduce their calories. Low-carb dieters will often see improvement in their insulin, blood sugar, and triglyceride levels.

The reason for this is the way in which your body works. When carbs are consumed, your body turns them into glucose, which raises your blood sugar. Your body then produces insulin to reduce your blood sugar levels. Years of this will cause your body to have to produce more insulin. This can cause you to become insulin resistant, which can turn into type 2 diabetes.

The ADA has found that one in three adults in the US are prediabetic, and one in ten have type 2 diabetes. CDC says that the number of obese adults in the US has spiked since the 1980s from 15% to 35% of people aged 20 to 74. This is largely due to a change in diet.

The USDA made their first dietary guideline release in 1980, and they said that fats and oils needed to be heavily reduced as well as sweets. They said that carbohydrates should make up the most of your daily food consumption. They soon released the Food Pyramid Guide, which put carbs at the bottom and recommended that you eat six to 11 servings a day. They also told us to eat two to four servings of fruit. Decades later, this guideline is still the framework for the US consumer education messages from various government organizations.

Healthy carbs are still suggested for diabetics instead of reducing carbs. If carbs are made up of mostly sugar, and sugar is what caused the disease, why should carbs be the main part of your diet? There are no essential carbohydrates. The body is able to create its own glucose through gluconeogenesis.

On the flip side, you have no doubt heard that monounsaturated and saturated fats cause heart disease among other health problems. In just the last decade, dozens of studies have found similar conclusions: these types of fats have no effect on heart disease risk.

The majority of fats are essential for our health; this is why we have essential fatty acids and essential amino acids. Fats are a more efficient form of energy and contain around nine calories. When the majority of your diet is made up of fats, your body will adapt and use stored fats for energy, but more on that later.

This book is here to provide you with the information that you need to succeed with a ketogenic diet through simple cooking to achieve long-term success and weight loss.

# Chapter 1: Low-Carb and High-Fat

The easiest way to explain the ketogenic diet is that it is a diet that is high in fats, low in carbohydrates, and a medium consumption of protein. This diet became a popular way to treat refractory epilepsy in children. This diet causes the body to burn fat rather than carbohydrates for its energy source.

The carbs that many people eat get converted into glucose. The body then transports it around, and it is important to fuel the brain. If our bodies don't have a lot of carbs, the liver will convert fats that have been stored in the body into ketone bodies and fatty acids. These ketones will go to the brain and replace the glucose. These raised ketones are what helps reduce the frequency of seizures related to epilepsy.

About half of the children who were put on this diet had a reduction in the number of seizures they had. The good news is the effects continue after they returned to their normal diet.

The classic keto diet will contain about a four to one ratio by weight of combined carbs and protein to fat. This can be done by getting rid of foods that are high in carbs such as pasta, sugar, bread, grains, fruits, and vegetables that are starchy. This diet also increases the consumption of cream, butter, and nuts that are high in fat.

Most of the fats that are found in foods are LCTs or long-chain triglycerides. What's crazy is that MCTs or medium-chain triglycerides are the ones who are more ketogenic. Many people who follow the ketogenic diet use coconut oil a lot because it is high in MCTs. They might also choose to buy MCT oil and put it in their coffee for an added boost each morning.

Every person's needs and body will be a bit different; what macros makeup in a normal keto diet is normally 60 to 75 percent of their calories will come from fat, 15 to 30 percent comes from protein, and five to ten percent are from carbs.

After you've been on the diet for a few days, your body enters what is called ketosis, but we will go into that later. This is when the body begins using the fat that has been stored and eating it for energy.

Even though this diet was created to treat epilepsy, people began noticing it was useful in losing weight. Basically, when you eat carbs, your body will retain fluid so it can store the carbs for energy. When you aren't consuming as many carbs, you will lose all the water that has been stored.

Most people who begin this diet want to lose weight. This diet is great for that because it gets rid of all the stored fat in the body.

This diet seems hard to stick with because it does restrict many foods, but there are many creative ways to ensure you don't miss out on tasty meals. If you can stick with it, you are going to notice your waistline beginning to shrink.

There are many foods out there that target keto dieters. FATBAR is the first one to come to mind. Their snack bars contain 200 calories, 16 grams of fat, and four net grams of carbs.

If you love coffee and love having a vanilla latte each morning, you can start drinking bulletproof coffee instead. This is normal coffee with some MCT oil and butter mixed in.

Being able to maintain a low-carb, high-fat diet is essential for weight loss. It helps reduce risk factors for Alzheimer's, stroke, heart diseases, diabetes, and more. This diet encourages you to eat whole foods such as healthy oils and fats, veggies, fish, and meat. It reduces all the chemically and processed foods. This diet is one you can keep doing long term and be able to enjoy it. Why can't you enjoy a diet that lets you eat eggs and bacon?

Carbs get turned into sugar when digested, and this causes crashes which will lead to cravings for carbs. This cycle will cause insulin spikes and could lead to prediabetes and type 2 diabetes.

Studies show that this diet can help people lose weight, improve their energy levels, and stay satiated for longer. This increased satiety and energy come from the calories you are getting from fats. These fats get digested slowly and are dense in calories. Dieters who follow this diet will consume fewer calories since they feel fuller longer and don't get hungry as often.

## Beginning a Keto Diet

Many people will shorten the ketogenic diet to just keto. The word keto is derived from the fact that your body will create fuel molecules called ketones. These get used as an alternative fuel source for the body when glucose is in short supply.

When you eat a few carbs, these ketones get produced. This holds true when you keep your protein intake to a moderate level. Too much protein can be turned into sugar.

The liver will create these ketones from the stored fat in your body. Our bodies will then use these ketones as fuel in different parts of the body along with the brain. The brain uses a lot of energy each day, but it can't fun off fat. It can only get energy through ketones or glucose.

When following a keto diet, your whole body will change its fuel supply to run almost completely on fat. Your insulin level will drop, and fat burning will increase. It will be easier for the body to access the fat stores in order to burn them. This is great when you want to lose weight. There are other benefits that aren't as obvious such as mental alertness, less hunger, and more energy.

## How Low is Low-Carb?

This diet works best when you consume very little carbs. The less you eat, the more effective it is going to be for you to lose weight. A keto diet is a very strict low-carb diet. You are going to consume about 20 grams or less of net carbs each day.

When you have reached your weight loss goals, you can begin to increase your carb intake. This needs to be done slowly, so you don't gain the weight back.

## Basics

This is a great diet; there is a right and wrong way to do it. You have to begin this diet the right way, so you get faster and better results.

On paper, the keto diet is fairly simple: you eat low carbs and high fat. This doesn't tell you what you can and can't eat. There is a complete list of foods that are fine to eat along with foods that are restricted later in the book, but here is a basic list of what you can have:

- Meats including organ meats
- Heavy fats like butter, lard, bacon fat, ghee, olive oil, coconut oil, and tallow
- Fish and seafood
- Eggs
- Certain berries such as raspberries, blueberries, and strawberries
- Vegetables that aren't starchy. You are going to want to eat all the leafy greens you can.

This means that the food you eat in a typical day might look like:

- Breakfast: eggs and bacon
- Lunch: a cup of bone broth and chicken salad
- Dinner: vegetables along with a steak and even a dessert that is ketogenic-friendly.

Some people can't go through their day without having a snack. This is fine as long as you stick with broth, cheese sticks, nuts, celery sticks, and meat sticks. You need to watch the snacks, you will have to add it into your total macros for the day.

The keto diet is easy to personalize it. You have the ability to experiment and see what is going to work best for you. Some people find they need more fats in their diet while others will be able to eat more carbs. Some people even try intermittent fasting.

Many people that intermittent fast will skip breakfast and will eat their first meal at about one in the afternoon. This will up your ketosis power.

## Macros

Macros have been mentioned before, and you might be wondering what they are. Macros are short for macronutrients when talking about the ketogenic diet.

Macros are parts of the food that gives you fuel and energy. These are protein, carbohydrates, and fats. These are what gives you your dietary calories. It's important that you totally understand what macros are if you want to succeed with this diet. These have to be in the correct balance for you to remain in ketosis.

Carbs are the only macros that you don't have to eat to be able to live. There are essential amino acids and fatty acids that are building blocks for fats and proteins, but carbohydrates aren't essential.

Carbs are made up of two things' sugars and starches. Fiber is looked at as a carb, but with the keto diet, it doesn't get counted into your total carb intake. Fiber isn't counted because your body doesn't digest fiber, so it doesn't affect your blood sugar.

When you look at a nutrition label on a food, you need to look at the total carb amount and then look at the fiber. You will need to subtract the total about of fiber from the total amount of carbs. This gives you your net carb amount.

Total carbs – fiber = net carbs

What this means is that net carbs only count the sugars and starches in the carbohydrates. What you are trying to figure your macros for your meals, you only use the net carbs. You don't have to use the total number of carbs.

In order to succeed, you need to find foods that are low in carbohydrates naturally and the ones that aren't. Not all of them are obvious. It is obvious that potatoes are high in carbs, but did you know that bananas are also high in carbs?

For people who are just beginning the keto diet, they should try to consume about 20 grams of net carbs every day.

Protein is important for the body since it helps keep lean muscle mass, a source of energy when carbs aren't available, makes hormones and enzymes, immune function, growth, and tissue repair. Protein has an important role in the body's biological process. Proteins are called the building blocks of a healthy body.

When we consume proteins, they get broken down into amino acids. Nine of these aren't able to be produced by the body. This is why we need to get these essential amino acids from the foods we eat. These nine essential amino acids are phenylalanine, valine, histidine, tryptophan, isoleucine, threonine, leucine, methionine, and lysine. Where there's a deficiency in protein or any of these amino acids, it could cause malnutrition, kwashiorkor, or many other health problems.

When you are following a ketogenic diet, you need to make sure you eat enough protein to preserve your lean body mass. The amount you consume depends on the amount of lean body mass you have right now. Here is a guideline:

- 0.7 to 0.8 grams of protein per pound of muscle to help preserve your muscle mass.

- 0.8 to 1.2 grams of protein per pound of muscle to increase your muscle mass.

You don't want to ever lose body mass. You need to aim to preserve or gain. Many people only focus on losing weight, but a lot of the time losing weight means losing muscle along with the fat. Your goal should be to lose fat and save your muscle. This is important for you to keep good metabolism.

The main thing to remember is not to go crazy when you eat protein while doing keto. Too much might end up putting stress on your kidneys, and this can affect ketosis. Aim to keep your macros in the above ranges.

Take a look at this example:

Let's say you weigh 160 pounds and you have a body fat percentage of 30 percent. This would mean you have about 48 pounds of body fat. Now you are going to subtract your body fat from your total weight. This gives you your lean body mass. For this example, it would be 112 pounds.

In order to figure out the amount of protein you need to eat, you need to take your lean body mass number and multiply by the ratio from earlier. For this example, you need to consume 89.6 grams of protein every day to preserve your muscle mass. It would look like this:

112 pounds muscle X .8 grams of protein = 89.6 grams

The last macro is fats. We need to consume a decent amount of fat to maintain cell membranes, provide cushioning for protecting the organs, absorbing specific vitamins, growth, energy, and development. These fats also help you feel fuller longer.

Dietary fats get broken down into fatty acids and glycerol. Our bodies can't synthesize two types of fatty acids, so we have to include them in our diets. These fatty acids are linolenic acid and linoleic acid.

These fats are sating, so it is perfect for anyone who is looking to help fight hunger pangs. Now all you have to do is figure out the amount of fat you need to eat. If your carbs are at the lowest possible, you know how much protein you need to consume, the rest of your dietary needs will have to be met with fat.

To maintain your weight, you need to eat enough calories from fat to support your normal expenditure. If you are wanting to burn fat, then you need to eat in the deficit.

You have been given a lot of information to help you find your macros, there are easier ways to figure this out. There are many online calculators to help you figure out these numbers without getting a headache. If you would like to use an online calculator, check out the website Ketogains. Theirs works great.

If you would like to see how figuring out for yourself will work, let's continue to use the 160-pound example from earlier. We're going to assume this person is a female, stands, 5' 4", in her late 20s and sits behind a desk all day. This means she is mostly sedentary.

Let's put her information into a calculator:

Base metabolic rate is 1467 kcal.

Daily energy expenditure would be 1614 kcal.

She is going to need to eat about 90 grams of protein, 20 grams of net carbs, and 86 grams of fat. Her intake is made up of 72 percent fat, 23 percent protein, and five percent carbs.

Now that you know what macros are and the way to figure your numbers, you are on your way to beginning the ketogenic diet.

## Why Try Keto?

When you are on a ketogenic diet, your body gets good at burning stored fat for its fuel. This is wonderful for many reasons, one of them is the fact that fat contains more calories than most carbs so you can eat less food each day. Your body will easily burn the stored fat, and this results in more weight that is lost. Using fat as fuel will provide constant levels of energy. It won't spike your blood sugar, and this means you won't experience the lows and high when eating carbs. Having constant levels of energy through your day means you will get more done and won't feel tired when doing it.

In addition to these benefits, following a keto diet can:

- Improves brain function
- Improves HDL (good) levels and LDL (bad) cholesterol
- Reduces blood pressure
- Reduces triglycerides
- Reduces insulin resistance and blood sugar. This can reverse prediabetes and type 2 diabetes.
- Results in loss of more body fat.

There are many different things that could happen when following a keto diet. Let's talk about some.

**Helps your brain focus**

A ketogenic diet helps increase your clarity, memory, cognition, fewer migraines, and seizure control. The first use of this diet was in the 1920s at the Mayo Clinic to help children who had epilepsy. The exact reason behind the prevention of seizures while doing a keto diet is still unknown, but scientist thinks it is because it causes more stability in the neurons and up-regulation of mitochondrial enzymes and brain mitochondria.

Close to this, there has been some attention given to this diet and how it affects Alzheimer's disease. Researchers found there was improved memory and increased cognition in adults who had problems in these areas. More research has found improvement with every stage of dementia. Ketosis can help fight Parkinson's disease.

For the larger audience of keto followers, there have been fewer side effects and less frequent migraines along with better mental clarity and focus. This is because of the more stable blood sugar and the change of chemistry in the brain that helps with memory and cognition.

## Cancer Fighter

Dom D'Agostino's lab figured out that ketone supplementation was able to decrease the viability of tumor cells and helped to prolong the life of mince that had metastatic cancer. Cancer cell metabolism works abnormally when compared to healthy cells. These get increased through consuming glucose because of genetic mutations and mitochondrial dysfunction. Some studies show that unlike healthy tissues, cancer cells can't use ketone bodies for energy. Ketones also inhibit the proliferation and viability of tumor cells.

This isn't saying that if you have cancer, you should stop your normal treatments. You should always follow your doctor's advice.

## Prevents Heart Disease

Following a keto diet could help lower blood pressure and triglycerides along with improving cholesterol. This happens because this diet keeps blood glucose low and stable. This might sound counterintuitive that eating fats will help you lower your triglycerides; it has been proven that eating too many carbs is the main reason behind high triglyceride levels.

When talking about LDL and HDL, the keto diet can help up HDL levels. This is the good cholesterol. It can also help to improve LDL profiles.

## Decreases Inflammation

In an article in Nature Medicine, it was found that the mechanism behind what has been believed for decades: a keto diet is anti-inflammatory and could help with many other issues.

Research has found that these might be connected to "BHB-mediate inhibition of the NLRP3 inflammasome."

This basically says that inflammatory diseases can be suppressed by BHB. This is a ketone that is produced with following a ketogenic diet. This has helped other problems like arthritis, eczema, IBS, acne, psoriasis, and other inflammatory diseases that have prompted more research.

## Improves Energy and Sleep

By the time people reach day four or five on the diet, many will report an increase in energy and fewer carb cravings. The main reason for this is stable insulin levels and a readily available energy source for the body tissues and brain.

It still isn't understood why it improves sleep. Studies have shown that the ketogenic diet helps with sleep because it decreases REM and increases slow-wave sleep patterns. The exact reason why is unclear. It has something to do with the complex biochemical shift involved with the brain using ketones for energy when combined with the body burning fat.

## Stable Uric Acid Levels

The main cause of kidney stones and gout is elevated levels of uric acid, calcium, phosphorus, and oxalate. This is due to the combination of consuming things with many purines and alcohol, obesity, sugar consumption, unlucky genetics, and dehydration.

There is a caveat though; a ketogenic diet will temporarily raise your uric acid levels, especially if you let yourself get dehydrated. With time, the levels will go back down.

## Assists Gastrointestinal and Gallbladder Health

This means you will have less gas and bloating, improved digestion, less heartburn and acid reflux, and less risk of gallstones.

It is known that sugary foods, nightshades such as potatoes and tomatoes, and grain-based foods can increase the chances of a person getting acid reflux and heartburn.

It shouldn't surprise you to learn that eating fewer carbs can improve these symptoms and confront the problems of bacterial issues, inflammation, and autoimmune responses.

A ketogenic diet will rapidly and reproducible alter our gut microbiome. Dr. Eric Westman explains how many problems are reduced or removed because of these microbiome changes.

Research has found that consuming carbs is one of the main causes of gallstones. When you eat enough fat while your intake of carbs is low, it will clear up gallbladders and make things run a lot more smoothly.

## Assists with Women's Health

One review published in 2013 looked at evidence of the ways a keto diet could enhance fertility. Research shows that PCOS can be treated effectively by following a low-carb diet. This can help reduce or eliminate symptoms such as acne, obesity, and infrequent or prolonged periods.

Basically, when you keep your blood sugar low and stable, it will help to stabilize and equilibrate other hormone levels. This can cause other benefits on a large array of metabolic pathways that get treated with insulin such as hunger and energy utilization.

## Helps the Eyes

The largest problems many diabetics face is macular degeneration. It is known that high blood sugar could hurt people's eyesight and might lead to greater risks of cataracts. It shouldn't surprise you that when you keep your blood sugar levels low, it can improve your vision health and improve your eyes.

## Help Muscle Gain and Improves Endurance

It has been found that BHB can help promote muscle gain. If you combine this with other evidence through the years, there has been an increase in the bodybuilder movement toward a keto approach to gain muscle.

Ultra-endurance athletes have turned to the keto diet, too. After the athlete has become completely fat-adapted, there is some evidence that suggests that their physical and mental performance will be improved.

## Improves Obesity, Diabetes, and Metabolic Syndrome

This is the main reason why people begin a ketogenic diet. For all the reasons we've covered, a keto diet is wonderful for people who have been diagnosed with type 1 or type 2 diabetes.

It can also be effective for obesity because it helps burn fat and prevents muscle loss. It can also prevent disorders that are related to obesity. This includes all of the symptoms and risk factors are known as metabolic syndrome.

# Chapter 2: Keto in Steps

Now that you know the science behind the ketogenic diet and the reasons it works, you are going to learn how to get started and how to maximize your success. Here is an easy and quick guide for you to use when starting. You can also look back over it anytime you need to in your journey when you need some guidance and support.

## Clean Out the Pantry

When you have unhealthy, tempting foods in your house, it is the largest contributor to failure when beginning any diet. In order to succeed, you have to get rid of any triggers if you want to maximize your chances. If you don't have the iron will of The Rock, you have to keep addictive foods such as desserts, bread, and any other non-keto-friendly snacks in your house.

If you live with others, you need to talk about what you are doing before you just throw out everything. If there are some things that you can throw away because they don't belong to you, try to find a location that will keep them out of your sight. This will let your roommates know that you are serious about your new lifestyle. It will lead to better experiences for you at home, too. Other people love to tempt others who are trying to diet when they begin, but they usually tire out quickly.

- Grains and Starches

Throw out all the croissants, rolls, wraps, bagels, bread, flour, quinoa, oats, corn, potatoes, rice, pasta, and cereal.

- Drinks and Sugary Foods

Throw out all candy bars, milk chocolate, pastries, desserts, milk, fruit juices, fountain drinks, and refined sugars.

- Legumes

Throw away all lentils, peas, and beans. These are dense with carbs. Just a one cup serving of beans will contain more than three times the number of carbs you need in one day.

- Processed Polyunsaturated Oils and Fats

Throw out all vegetable oils and most oils that are made from seeds like corn, grapeseed, soybean, canola, safflower, and sunflower. Try to get rid of any trans fats such as margarine and shortening. Basically, anything that says "partially hydrogenated" or "hydrogenated." Coconut, avocado, extra-virgin olive, and olive oil are the only oils you need to keep on hand.

- Fruits

Throw away all fruits that are high in carbs like apples, mangos, grapes, dates, and bananas. Make sure to throw out any dried fruits such as raisins. Fruits that have been dried contains the same amount of sugar as the regular fruit, but it is more concentrated. This makes it easy to eat too much sugar in just one small serving. Look at this comparison: one cup of raisins will have over 100 grams of carbs while a cup of grapes will only have 15 grams of carbs.

You might be "throwing out" your unwanted foods, but this food could feed others. Don't just chuck them in the garbage, donate them to a local food pantry to help feed the homeless.

Your pantry is going to look empty after you have cleaned it out. This is because products that are meant to be stored long term are full of unhealthy additives, preservatives, and carbs. We are going to fill your refrigerator in the next step.

## Let's Go Shopping

Now it is time to restock your freezer, refrigerator, and pantry with keto-friendly, delicious foods that will make you feel great, get healthy, and lose weight.

- Basics

When you have these basics on hand, you will be able to prepare keto-friendly, delicious, and healthy snacks and meals.

- Seeds and nuts like pumpkin seeds, chia seeds, flaxseed, pine nuts, hazelnuts, walnuts, almonds, pecans, and macadamia nuts.
- Fermented and pickled foods such as sauerkraut, kimchee, and pickles.
- Broths like bone, beef, and chicken.
- Low-carb condiments such as Sriracha, pesto, mustard, and mayonnaise.
- Lime or lemon juice
- Sweeteners like erythritol and stevia
- Any herbs and spices your heart desires
- Tea, coffee, and water
- Meats

Any meat is fine for this diet including wild game, turkey, pork, lamb, beef, and chicken. It is preferred to use organic or grass-fed meats if they are readily available and you can afford them. You should and can eat the fat on the meat and the skin of the chicken.

All wild-caught seafood and fish goes well with the keto diet very well. Try to stay away from any farm-raised fish.

You can have all the eggs you would like. Use free-range or organic eggs if at all possible.

- Vegetables

You are allowed to eat all the vegetables that aren't starchy like cauliflower, Summer squash, zucchini, olives, eggplant, Brussels sprouts, garlic (in limited quantities – every clove contains one gram of carbs), tomatoes, peppers, onions, lettuce, cucumbers, mushrooms, asparagus, and broccoli.

Stay away from all kinds of potatoes, sweet potatoes, yams, corn. Avoid legumes such as peas, lentils, and beans.

- Fruits

You can have a small number of berries each day like blueberries, blackberries, raspberries, and strawberries. Lime and lemon juice is great to add flavor to meals. Avocados are full of healthy fats and are very low in carbs.

Stay away from all other fruits since they are loaded with sugars. One banana contains about 25 grams of net carbs.

- Dairy

You need to eat full-fat dairies such as unsweetened yogurt, cream cheese, cheese, heavy cream, sour cream, and butter. It isn't technically dairy, unsweetened coconut and almond milk are great to have, too.

Stay away from skim milk, sweetened yogurt, and milk because they contain sugar. Stay away from all fat-free, low fat, or any flavored dairy products.

- Oils and Fats

Bacon fat, lard, butter, olive oil, and avocado oil are great for eating and cooking. Avocado oil has a high smoke point which is great for searing meats and frying in a wok. A high smoke point oil means the oil won't smoke or burn until it hits 520 degrees Fahrenheit. Be sure to stay away from oils that have been labeled "blend." These will contain small amounts of healthy oils and add in large amounts of unhealthy oils.

## Setting up The Kitchen

Preparing recipes is the best part of the ketogenic diet, and it is very easy when you have the correct tools. These tools will make cooking faster and easier. Each one is worth the money especially if you cook a lot.

- ***Food Scale***

When you are trying to hit your macro and calorie goals, a food scale is completely necessary. You will be able to measure any liquid or solid food. You will get the correct amount each time. If you use it along with an app such as "MyFitnessPal," you will have all the information you need to hit your goals. You can find food scales online for around ten to 20 dollars.

- *Food Processor*

These little beauties are essential for your kitchen. These are great for blending or processing foods together to make shakes and sauces. Blender just won't cut it, for most foods like cauliflower and other tough vegetables.

One great food processor/blender is the Nurtibullet. The container you blend with has lids and drink spouts so you can make a shake and take it with you. They are easy to clean, and this makes the entire system very convenient. You can usually find these for around $80 online.

- *Vegetable Spiralizer*

These cute little things will turn vegetable into ribbons or noodles in just seconds. They make cooking easier and faster. Noodles have more surface area and don't take as long to cook. A spiralizer can turn zucchini into noodles. Just add some marinara or Alfredo sauce, and you will never know you are eating zucchini. These cost about $30 and can either be found online or in retail stores.

- *Electric Hand Mixer*

If you have ever tried to beat an egg white by hand until stiff peaks form, you know how hard it can be. Electric mixers will save your arms and time, especially if you are mixing heavy ingredients. You can find good ones anywhere for around $10 to $20.

- *Cast Iron Pans*

These have been around for hundreds of years and were one of the very first modern cooking devices. Cast iron skillets won't wear out and are healthier for you since they don't contain any chemicals. They retain heat extremely well and can be taken off the stove and put straight into the oven. They are easy to clean. Just wipe them out with a non-scratchy sponge, dry them, and rub them down with cooking oil before you put them away. This will prevent them from rusting and will help season them. You will soon have a natural nonstick surface. When you buy a new cast iron pan, most will come pre-seasoned, and this preserves the coating. You can find them in any retail store or online from between $10 and $80. It all depends on the size and brand. The lodge is the most popular brand, and it is made in the United States.

- *Knife Sharpening Stone*

The majority of your prep time will be spent cutting foods. You will see your cutting speed skyrocketed with a set of sharp knives. It is fun to use sharp knives. Try to sharpen your knives each week to keep them in tip-top shape. Sharpening stones usually cost less than $10. They can be found in most retail stores or online.

# Exercise

When you exercise more, you are going to have better health. If you follow a keto diet, you are going to lose weight quickly and improve your health. What happens when you combine the two?

I would be easy to assume that combining the two will take your health and weight loss to new levels, but the truth is a bit more complicated. With the restriction of carbs, there is a lot of change that could happen, and some of these will affect how well you exercise.

With the restricted carb intake, you are limiting your muscles from getting sugar, which is the easiest fuel source. When your muscles can't access sugar, their high-intensity function will be impaired. High intensity is any activity that lasts longer than ten seconds. The reason for this is that, after ten seconds of max effort, the muscles will produce energy from glucose through a metabolic pathway called as glycolysis. Glycolysis happens rather than the process in the phosphagen system.

Fat and ketones are not good substitutes for glucose during this time. After you have been exercising for two minutes, your body will shift into a metabolic pathway that will use fat and ketones.

Basically, when you are restricting your carb intake, you deprive the cells of your muscles of sugar that they need to fuel activities for high-intensity efforts for ten seconds to two minutes. This means if you are following a keto diet, it is going to limit your performance during exercises such as:

- Playing a sport that gives you minimal breaks like soccer, rugby, and lacrosse.
- Weight lifting for more than five reps each set using a weight that is heavy enough to almost cause you to fail.
- Interval training or high-intensity circuit training
- Sprinting or swimming for more than ten seconds.

This list is not comprehensive, but it will give you an idea of the types of exercises that your body uses glycolysis for. Remember that the metabolic pathway timing varies on each individual. There are people who have the capacity to maintain performance for 30 seconds without needing any carbs at all.

It is important for you to consume the correct amount of fat and protein when exercising and doing keto.

Many health professionals, when they design a diet plan, will arrange the protein intake first. This is because protein always gets top priority as it performs many actions that carbs and fats can't. Protein will help improve satiation, has a better thermic effect, and stimulates muscles synthesis better than all the other macronutrients. If enough protein isn't consumed, you will lose muscle mass and might end up eating more calories.

If you are going to keep your exercise regimen or begin one, which you really should, you need to make sure you eat the correct amount of macros. Here are some guidelines:

- The majority of your excess calories should come from fat and not protein or carbs.

- Keep the protein intake to one gram per pound of body weight.

- Be sure your calorie intake stays around a deficit of 250 to 500 calories. This is not a top priority. Many people don't worry about calories all the much when doing a keto diet.

Now that you have to be careful and smart with eating while exercising, let's learn some exercises that are good with keto.

## Keto Along with Cardio

The good thing for most of us is we aren't athletes so adding an exercise routine won't be hard. Cardio workouts don't require you to exercise intensively to require your body to burn glycogen and sugar for you to see the results. You just have to work to bring your heart rate up and keep it there.

Because cardio is a low to moderate intensity exercise, a keto diet won't impair your performance. You might realize that you have the ability to work out for a longer time without tiring as quickly when you are in ketosis.

The intensity you need to aim for in order to get the most out of your workout is moderate intensity. When you aim for moderate-intensity physical activity, you should get your heart rate to 50 to 70 percent of your max heart rate.

In order for you to estimate your max heart rate, begin by subtracting your age from 220. If you are 50 years old, to figure out your age-related heart rate, you would take 220 and subtract 50. This gives you 170 beats per minute. This you can figure out the 50 to 70 percent levels, which would be:

- 70 percent – 170 x 0.70 = 119

- 50 percent – 170 x 0.50 = 85

This means that a 50-year-old person, in order to partake in moderate=intensity physical activity, you need to keep your heart between 85 and 119 beats per minute.

When you set out yourself to keep a ketogenic diet, your objective should be to aim for the bottom end of the range. When you have been on the diet for a couple of weeks, you will begin to see that you can maintain a higher heart rate without needing any extra carbs.

If you are new to working out and cardio, you want to stick to 50 percent if your max heart rate for around ten to 15 minutes. You can begin increasing the duration by five or so every week until you can work out for 30 to 45 minutes at 50 percent of your max heart rate. When you have managed to do this, you can start increasing your intensity level every week until you have reached 70 percent of your max heart rate.

If you aren't sure what works best for cardio workouts, here are some examples:

- Cycling
- Aerobic training classes
- Running
- Swimming
- Circuit training
- Recreational sports
- Interval training classes

You need to remember that your strength and power might become decreased during these workouts due to carb restriction. If you just want to get a good cardio workout, then it isn't important that you push yourself to the max for your strength and power.

This isn't saying that you can't increase your strength and power while on a keto diet. All you need to do to achieve this is practice mindful exercising.

## Keto and Weight Lifting

You can increase power, muscle mass, and strength when following a ketogenic diet. The best thing to do is improve all these at the same time by using the same program.

It was stated earlier that without glucose your body could only last for ten seconds with high-intensity exercises. This means if you are a weightlifter you could improve strength and power, as well as muscle mass by doing sets that won't last longer than ten seconds.

This means if you follow a program that requires five or more sets of five or fewer reps for every exercise, then this is great for people who follow a ketogenic diet.

Some research has found that lower reps might be helpful when talking about hypertrophy. This means that your muscles don't need you to pump out eight to 12 reps in a row to get bigger. What your muscles are looking for is the correct amount of volume, this depends on the person, and for your volume to increase every week.

This means that you can build muscles without carbs. Carbohydrates might be needed for some high-intensity work, but a bodybuilder doesn't have to eat a lot of carbs to see any results.

## Exercise and Keto in Harmony

In order to mix these two things, you need to make the correct changes to your workout program and diet so that you don't cause any adverse reactions, especially if you do high-intensity workouts.

When you try to add in exercise just to improve your health, then you can experiment with things a bit more than an athlete can. In general, you need to try lifting weights and cardio training each week. Cardio needs to be done two to three times every week, and you need to lift weights two or three times every week. You don't need to try to do both of these on the same day.

# Chapter 3: What to Expect

The ketogenic diet is safe and effective there are some dangers and downsides. Before we go into the dangers, let's look at some side effects that you might experience when you finally enter ketosis.

## Side Effects of Keto

Not all the side effects of keto are bad, but there are a few that can be definitely unpleasant.

- *You might feel tired or sick*

You might have heard people talk about the keto flu. This is totally real. When you cut carbs and enter into ketosis, it can cause many uncomfortable symptoms like muscle aches, diarrhea, headaches, nausea, and fatigue. These side effects are caused by your body transitioning into learning to use fat as its source of energy instead of using carbs. When your body has finally adapted to this new fuel source, which will take about a week or two, you will notice that you begin to feel better.

- *You might lose weight fast, but it could come back*

Ketogenic diets are popular because of the fast slim down. This is because your body releases a lot of water when your body begins using fat for energy. Your scales will go down a few pounds, and you might even look leaner.

That first drop you experience will probably only be water weight. This isn't saying you haven't burned off any fat. The problem is, while studies have shown that you are going to lose weight, they haven't figured out if it can be sustained long-term. Many people find that a strict eating plan is tough to stick with. If you go off the diet, you might gain back all the weight.

- *You might feel less hungry*

Many diets are associated with feeling hungry and constantly fighting off cravings. This isn't necessarily true with the keto diet. There are many people who say they aren't as hungry and don't feel like eating all the time. Researchers aren't clear as to why this happens, but they believe that low-carb diets suppress ghrelin which is a hunger that controls hunger.

- *You will feel very thirsty*

Don't worry if you begin to feel parched when following a keto diet. You are going to be expelling a lot of water, and it is going to spike your thirst. Be sure you drink a lot of water. There isn't a set amount, but you need to drink enough so that your urine is clear to pale yellow.

- *Your acne could clear up*

If you have always been bothered with acne, you might find that the keto diet might clear it up. This is especially true if you always ate a lot of sugar. Empty carbs are the worst for acne since they trigger inflammation. Studies have shown that curbing your carb intake might fix these problems.

- *Not as much brain fog*

Everyone knows that carbs especially refined ones such as sugar, white bread, and white paste can cause your blood sugar to dip and spike. It is easy to see why eating less of them will keep your blood sugar steady. For people who are generally healthy, this means you will have a steady flow of energy, fewer cravings for sugar, and not as much brain fog.

- *Your A-1C levels might get better*

If you have diabetes, having better control of your blood sugar might help you control you're a-1C. It might even reduce your need for insulin. This isn't saying you need to stop taking your meds. The main downside is that it could up your risk of developing diabetic ketoacidosis which is life-threatening. This is more common in people who have type 1 diabetes. If you have type 2, you should still speak with your doctor first before beginning any diet.

- *Low levels of energy*

This is normal while your body is adjusting to the switch in fuel sources. Good news for you is after your body gets adjusted your energy levels will improve.

## Dangers of Keto

Now that you know some of the side effects that the keto diet might cause, and you know not to worry. The negative ones will usually go away when your body has adjusted to this diet. The following are something that might happen to you on the keto diet that might not be temporary. These are extremely rare, but the might happen.

- *Low blood sugar*

Most of the time, when you have reached ketosis, you will notice your blood sugar levels will be more stable and lower. This is why low-carb diets are effective at controlling type 2 diabetes. Monitoring your carbs has been used for some time now as a way to control blood sugar. One study found that diets low in carbs isn't any better for long-term control than other diets.

There is some anecdotal evidence that says people who are diabetic with type 2 diabetes were actually able to stop taking their medicine because they were able to stabilize their blood sugar. This is not recommended, and if you have diabetes, please talk with your doctor first.

During the first few days, while the body is adapting to change, your body is going to be in a constant struggle with itself. You will need to ease into this diet if you are diabetic. Slowly cut back on the carbs otherwise you might cause your blood sugar to drop too much.

- *Nutritional deficiencies*

A diet that is high in fat and low in carbs will limit the types of foods that you can eat, and some complete food groups get eliminated altogether. Legumes, beans, and grains are all out along with many fruits and vegetables. Many of these foods carry nutrients, minerals, and vitamins that you can't get anywhere else. Without these foods, you might end up experiencing nutritional deficiencies.

Keto isn't a good idea for the long term since it isn't a completely balanced diet. Diets that don't allow fruits and vegetables will cause micronutrient deficiencies that could cause other consequences. It is great for short term fat loss, but it is best under the supervision of a medical professional.

- *Constipation and bowel changes*

When you eliminate fruits and vegetables from your diet, you won't be getting the nutrients you need, and it could cause other problems, too. These are the fiber-rich foods that will keep you regular. Without these foods, you might find that you are beginning to have changed with your bowels. This might include difficulty with bowel movements and possible constipation.

You need to be sure your load up on low-carb, fiber-rich foods such as cabbage, broccoli, and asparagus along with fats such as coconut oil and ghee.

- *Losing electrolytes*

After you have hit ketosis, your body is going to begin dumping stores of glycogen that is found in your fat and muscles that carry extra weight. This is going to make you use the bathroom more and could lead to electrolyte loss. Electrolytes are important for proper cardiac function and regular heartbeats. This might cause you to get cardiac arrhythmia.

Try to add electrolytes through natural sources or with OTC supplements.

- *Decreased serum sodium*

Normal Americans tend to consume too much salt, but when you are doing a keto diet, they might struggle to get enough. Low sodium can cause confusion, leg cramps, decreased energy, and vomiting. Be sure you add salt to every meal. Sea salt is best since it contains trace minerals.

- *Dehydration*

This is more common for people that are just beginning the keto diet since ketosis flushes your body of water. To prevent dehydration, it is best to aim for 2.5 liters of water every day. This should begin as soon as you begin this diet. You don't need to wait until you feel side effects.

- ***Kidney stones and kidney damage***

If you don't take care of your dehydration, it might cause acute kidney injury. But, that isn't the only way you could hurt your kidneys with the ketogenic diet. Excess protein could create high nitrogen levels that increase the pressure on the kidneys. This could cause kidney stones and can damage your kidney cells.

- ***Muscle loss***

The longer you keep your body in ketosis the more fat it is going to burn. The bad news is that you could lose muscle tissue, too. Yes, protein does help build muscle and is the powerhouse. Your muscles need carbs for formation and maintenance. Without carbs, the body might begin to break down your muscles.

- ***Heart problems***

Losing some heart muscle isn't the only risk associated with the heart that can happen while following the keto diet. If you already take medication for high blood pressure and you follow the keto diet, you might end up with abnormally low blood pressure results. If you have a heart condition, speak with your doctor before beginning the keto diet.

# Chapter 4: Ketosis and Reaching It

You've read the word ketosis numerous times in this book. Let's find out exactly what it is. Ketosis is a natural state your body goes into when it becomes fueled by fat. This will happen when a person fasts, or when they follow a strict low-carb diet.

There are many benefits for being in ketosis like health, performance, and weight loss. Remember that being in ketosis can have some side effects. For people who have type 1 diabetes and other diseases, excessive ketosis can become dangerous.

When you are in ketosis, your body will produce ketones. These are small fuel molecules, and our bodies use them as alternative fuel sources when glucose is in short supply. The liver will begin converting fat into ketones that get released into the bloodstream. The body can use them just like glucose. Our brains can also use the ketones as fuel, too.

## Getting into Ketosis

There are two ways our bodies can reach ketosis: by fasting or following a ketogenic diet. Under either of these circumstances, when the body's limited amount of glucose gets depleted, the body will switch its fuel source to fat. Insulin which is a fat storing hormone will get low and the body's ability to burn fat increases. This means your body has easy access to your stored fat and is able to get rid of them.

You can consider yourself in ketosis after your body makes enough ketones to make a significant level in the blood, usually more than 0.5 mM. The fastest way for this to happen is fasting, but you can't do that forever.

This is why people follow the keto diet since it can be eaten for an indefinite amount of time.

## Fuel for the Brain

Many people think you need carbs to fuel the brain. The brain will happily burn carbs when you eat them, but if carbs aren't available, it will eat ketones just as happily.

This is needed for basic survival. Because our bodies can only store carbs for one or two days, the brain would shut down after just a few days without food. Alternatively, it needs to quickly convert muscle protein into glucose, which isn't very effective, just to keep it working. This means we would waste away extremely fast. If this was how our bodies actually worked, then the human race would not have been able to survive before food became available 24/7.

Our bodies have evolved to work a lot smarter than that. Normally our bodies have stored fat that will last so we could survive for many weeks without food. Ketosis is the process that happens to make sure the brain can run on stored fat.

## Ketosis versus Ketoacidosis

There are many misconceptions about ketosis. The main one is mixing ketosis with ketoacidosis. Ketoacidosis is a rare and dangerous condition that will normally happen to people who have type 1 diabetes. There are many health care professionals who mix these two words up, too. It could be because their names are similar and there is a lack of knowledge between the differences.

Ketosis is a natural state that happens to the body, and the body is in total control of itself. Ketoacidosis is a malfunction of the body where it creates excessive amounts of ketones that the body can't regulate. This can cause things such as nausea, stomach pain, and vomiting this is then followed by confusion and coma. This requires urgent medical treatment and might end up being fatal.

Ketoacidosis will happen when ketones reach a level of 10 millimolar or more. People who follow a ketogenic diet will normally reach a level of three millimolar or less. There are many people who struggle to reach 0.5. Long-term starvation, which happens you have gone without food for 7 or more days, this could bring the number up to six or seven. Ketoacidosis might happen at level ten, but it normally happens around 15 and above.

The difference between these two things is like drinking a glass of water versus drowning in the ocean. Both of these things deal with water, but they are nowhere near being the same thing.

If you have a properly functioning pancreas that produced insulin which basically means you haven't been diagnosed with type 1 diabetes, it is going to be extremely hard for you to hit ketoacidosis even if you tried to. The reason for this is your body will release insulin when your body produces too many ketones, which shuts down ketone production.

## Getting to Optimal Ketosis

This is the state everyone who follows the keto diet wants to get to. Once you reach optimal ketosis, your body will burn fat at the fastest speed possible. In order to get to this optimal ketosis level, you have to follow a low-carb high-fat diet as stated above and keep your macros at the optimal level. There aren't any tricks to help you reach this level. There are some things that you can do.

Here are the different ketone levels you could have:

- Below 0.5 means you aren't in ketosis.

- Between 0.5 and 1.5 is a light level of nutritional ketosis. You will be losing weight, but it isn't at an optimal range.

- Around 1.5 to 3 is the optimal ketosis level and is the best for maximum weight loss.

- Levels over 3 aren't needed. High levels aren't going to help you one way or the other. It could harm you since it means that you aren't getting enough food.

There are many people who think they are eating a strict keto diet but end up being surprised when they measure their blood ketone levels. When they measure their blood, they end up being about 0.2 or 0.5, which is nowhere near that sweet spot.

The trick to getting past this plateau is you have to make sure you stay away from obvious sources of carbs but make sure your protein intake doesn't go higher than the fat intake. It was said before that protein won't change your glucose levels as carbs do, but if you do eat too many, especially if they exceed your fat intake, it will change your glucose. This is going to compromise your optimal ketosis level.

The secret to getting around this problem is to eat more fat. You can easily do this by adding a large dollop of herbed butter on top of your steak. This might keep you from eating too much or even eating seconds.

Drinking a cup of bulletproof coffee could also help you with hunger pangs and keep you from eating too much protein. This is easy as all you have to do is add a tablespoon of butter and a tablespoon of coconut oil to your morning coffee.

When you eat more fat, you will feel fuller. This makes sure you don't eat too much protein, and this helps you eat fewer carbs. This will help you reach an optimal level of ketosis.


## How to Measure Ketosis

There are several ways to figure out if you have reached ketosis. The first way is to measure ketones in your blood. This means you will have to purchase a meter and requires you to prick your finger.

There are several reasonably priced gadgets out there that will help you do this, and it will only take a few seconds to figure out what your blood ketone level is. Many people won't go to this extreme to figure out what their ketone level is, but this is the most accurate and effective.

You need to measure your blood ketones first thing every morning and on a fasted stomach. You can follow the levels that were listed earlier in this chapter to find out if you are in ketosis.

These meters will measure the amount of BHB that is in your blood. This is the main ketone that is present when you are in ketosis. The biggest downside of using this method is you have to draw blood.

Getting a test kit costs about $30 to $40 and might cost an extra $5 for each test. This is the main reason why people who choose this test will only test once each week or only every other week.

Okay, let's say you don't want to spend out more money on a blood ketone meter. Here are nine options that will help you figure out if you are in ketosis:

- *Ketones in breath and urine*

If you don't like the thoughts of pricking your finger, you can measure blood ketones by using a breath analyzer. This will check for acetone, which is one of the three ketones that will be present in your blood when you have reached ketosis.

This lets you know when you ketone levels have hit ketosis since acetone will leave the body when you reach nutritional ketosis. Breath analyzers are very accurate but not as accurate as monitoring your blood.

Another way you can check for ketosis is to check for ketones in the urine each day using special strips. This is a cheap and quick method to use to assess what your ketone levels are each day. These aren't extremely reliable methods though.

- *Bad breath*

This doesn't sound very pleasant, but many people have said that they have noticed bad breath once they have hit ketosis. This is a very common side effect. People say that their breath seems fruitier.

The reason for this is the elevated ketone levels. The main culprit is the ketone acetone that the body excretes through urine and breath. While you might not like the idea of having bad breath, it is a great way to know you are in ketosis. Many people will brush their teeth more often or chew sugar-free gum.

- *Weight loss*

This is probably the most obvious way to know you are in ketosis. When you first begin a keto diet, you will lose some weight very fast, but this is normally water weight. When you experience another drop in weight, which will be your fat stores. This is how you will know that you are in ketosis.

- *Better focus and energy*

Many people will sometimes report feeling tired, sick or having brain fog when they begin a keto diet. This is called the keto flu, but people who follow this for a long time reports increased focus and better energy. Your body needs to take time to adapt to this new diet. When you hit ketosis, your brain begins burning ketones for energy, and this might take a week or two to begin happening.

Ketones are a more potent fuel source for the brain when compared to carbs. This means it will improve your brain function and mental clarity.

- *Appetite suppression*

Many people say their hunger decreases when they begin following a keto diet. The reason behind this is still being researched. However, it is thought that the reduction in hunger is due to the increase in protein and vegetable consumption along with the change in your hunger hormones. The ketones might affect the way your brain reacts to hunger.

- *Digestive issues*

With all the major changes to the foods you are eating, you might experience some constipation or diarrhea when you first start this diet. This lets you know that you have almost reached ketosis. When the transition period is over, these problems should go away.

- *Short-term fatigue*

When your body begins making the switch into ketosis, it could cause weakness and fatigue, this makes it hard for some people to stick with the diet. This is a normal side effect but it lets you know you are hitting ketosis.

This crappy feeling might last for one week to one month before you fully hit ketosis, but in order to help reduce this feeling, you can take an electrolyte supplement.

- *Performance decrease*

Just like the point above, the fatigue could cause a slight decrease in exercise performance. This is because of the reduction in your muscle glycogen stores. This is what normally provides you with the fuel you need for your high-intensity workouts. After a week or two, your performance levels should return to normal.

- *Insomnia*

The biggest issue that many keto followers have is insomnia, especially when they first begin this diet. When your carbs become drastically reduced, it could cause some problems with sleeping. But, just remember that this, too, shall pass.

There are many different symptoms and signs that will tell you if you are in ketosis and if you are doing the right things. Ultimately, if you follow the rules for a keto diet and you stay consistent, your body will be in some form of ketosis.

If you want to know absolutely for certain if you are or aren't in ketosis, the best way to do this is by using a blood ketone monitor.

# Chapter 5: What Type is Right for You

Now that you know all the positive and negative aspects of this diet, it is time to decide which diet would work best for you. Yes, there is more than one type of keto diet. To make sure that you get the most from it, you should pick the diet that will work best for your health goals and needs. Every type will work best for various types of lifestyles.

## Four Kinds of Keto

There are four different types of ketogenic diets that you could follow depending on your life goals.

Here is one example, if you lead an active lifestyle or you are an athlete who likes doing high-intensity training, there is one keto diet that will be perfect for you. If you just want to lose some fat and reach our best healthy, there is one that will be perfect for you, as well.

- The standard ketogenic diet – fat loss and therapeutic purposes.
- Targeted ketogenic diet – workout performance.
- Cyclical ketogenic diet – bodybuilders and athletes.
- High-protein ketogenic diet – high protein needs.

Every one of these diets has their own rules, and they differ in the number of net carbs you get to eat every day.

## Standard Ketogenic Diet

This is the best option for beginners and anyone who wants to lose body fat, and for people who want to follow it for insulin resistance and therapeutic purposes.

You will begin eating 20 or fewer net carbs each day, and for the remainder of your diet is made up of 75 percent fats and 20 to 25 percent protein.

This is the most common ketogenic diet and is probably the best one to begin with if you haven't ever followed a keto diet before. This is the diet that is used to describe what the keto diet is and works best for most people.

The rules for the standard diet are:

- 20 grams of net carbs every day. Some resources tell you that you could actually eat up to 50 grams of carbs, but if you want to reach ketosis, you have to eat 30 or fewer grams daily.

- A decent amount of protein usually about .8 grams per pound of lean muscles mass.

- High amount of fat intake.

## Targeted Ketogenic Diet

This version is for people who know their bodies extremely well when it is ketosis and people who want to have extra energy for their exercise routines.

Your net carb intake is going to be about 20 to 50 fewer grams each day, normally 30 minutes to one hour before exercising. This is great for athletes who are very active.

This type of keto diet is targeted specifically to give you energy for workouts. Targeted refers to eating just after or before your workout times. This type of keto is best for people who know their limits and want the push themselves out of ketosis. This is great when you want to maintain exercise performance and lets glycogen re-synthesis happen without interrupting ketosis.

When you follow the targeted diet, you need to eat about 20 to 50 grams of net carbs in the hour right before you begin your workout. This is the number of carbs that will make up your day.

This diet is best for people who don't need to carb load, like people who follow a cyclical ketogenic diet and for people who don't want to exert any energy that would be needed to get the most out of a cyclical diet.

The best kinds of carbs to eat for the targeted diet are high on the glycemic index since these can be easily digestible. You need to aim for foods that are high in glucose and try to avoid fructose. Fructose gives the liver the glycogen it needs instead of creating glycogen from muscles which is what the keto diet tries to avoid.

This helps to avoid ketosis being disturbed since the carbs will be burned quickly and effectively during your workout. If you are eating the majority of your carbs close to the time of your workouts, you will need to watch for hidden carbs.

Both the targeted and cyclical diets are used for high-intensity exercise, but just because you are an athlete or lead an active lifestyle doesn't mean you have to follow either one of these keto diets.

Eating extra carbs has been recommended for active people or who perform high-intensity exercise regularly; however, there is some research that shows this isn't necessarily the case.

## Cyclical Ketogenic Diet

This is the best type for athletes, bodybuilders, and people who have done a keto diet before.

For this diet, you will eat a low number of net carbs for five to six days a week. Then you will eat a higher number of carbs for the other days of the week, and this cycles just repeats. People who absolutely have to eat carbs need to follow this diet.

The cyclical diet works along the lines of intermittent fasting that is followed with the 5/2 style of fasting since it has up and down days. The cyclical diet involves eating a keto diet for the majority of the week and then followed by a day or two of eating high carbs. These days are called carb-loading days.

Carb-loading involves alternating days of a keto diet with high-carb consumption days. These high-carb days might be 24 to 48 hours long. Normally, a cyclical diet requires you to consume about 50 grams of net carbs each day during the first phase, and then 150 to 200 grams of net carbs during the last phase.

Just like the targeted diet, a cyclical diet is best for people who understand their limits and can't break through their boundaries without some carb consumption.

This is best for athletes and bodybuilders who want to maximize their fat loss while building their lean muscle mass.

For advanced athletes who perform high volume and high-intensity exercises would be the biggest advantage for this keto diet. The goal of the cyclical diet is to deplete your muscle glycogen between your carb loading while a targeted diet has a goal of keeping your muscle glycogen at a moderate level.

## High Protein Ketogenic Diet

This type of ketogenic diet is best for people who want to follow the standard diet but wants or needs to eat more protein.

This works pretty much exactly like the standard ketogenic diet, except you eat more grams of protein every day. This means that instead of eating 5 percent carbs, 70 percent fats, and 25 percent protein, you will be eating 5 percent carbs, 60 percent fats, and 35 percent protein. This is great for anyone who lifts weights four to six days a week.

Even though you will be eating more protein with this diet, it isn't going to be enough to cause your blood sugar level to go up and knock you out of ketosis. One large myth that circles around this diet are that if you consume too much protein, it is going to knock you out of ketosis because of gluconeogenesis.

The process of GNG is very stable. You can't cause the rate of GNG to increase even if you eat extra protein. GNG is the process of making glucose from non-carbs, but it won't work at the rate as carb metabolism.

When someone eats chocolate cake, it is going to make their blood glucose to spike because of all the sugar in a very small window of time. When someone eats more protein, it isn't going to cause a spike in your blood sugar since the GNG is going to stay stable.

## Muscle Maintenance

If you are worried about losing muscle mass while following the ketogenic diet, your body has mechanisms that will help with muscle growth and maintenance while following this diet.

The ketones that the liver makes for energy contains protein-sparing properties, which prevents your muscles from breaking down. This is called beta-hydroxybutyrate or BHB.

Adrenaline plays a role in preserving muscle mass while in ketosis. When you have a drop in blood sugar, your body sends out a signal to produce adrenal secretions. Researchers have found that this secretion will help regular muscle mass by adrenergic influences.

This means that when the blood glucose drops due to a decrease in the intake of carbs, your body will send a signal to the adrenal glands that tell it to release epinephrine. Muscle proteins are greatly affected by these types of influences because of their hormonal activity that inhibits muscle breakdown.

This takes us back to the high protein diet. This diet, as stated above, have you eat more protein than is normally recommended for ketosis. When you eat an adequate amount of protein, it helps you maintain muscle mass.

While it appears that you are eating low amounts of protein, remember that when your body has become keto-adapted, it is going to use ketones and fats for energy which allows it to depend on these for fuel instead of protein.

## How to Choose the Right Diet

There isn't a straight forward answer to this question. The "calories in versus calories out" rule will only work to an extent. When this is followed, it doesn't think about what you are burning, lean mass or body fat.

While it might seem simple, meaning it doesn't matter what you are eating as long as you expend more than you take in, there are still other variables that haven't been put into play.

You, you are going to lose weight when you eat at a calorie deficit, but some of the weight you are losing could come from muscle. Research has found that even though you are consuming 15 to 25 percent of protein while doing the keto diet, you can eat at a calorie deficit while in ketosis without burning muscle mass.

If you are a beginner, it would be best for you to begin with the standard ketogenic diet. This allows your body to adjust to the diet in the easiest and quickest way and will make the transitioning into ketosis a lot easier.

Even if you are active, an athlete, starting with the standard keto diet will help guarantee the change in metabolism so that you won't need to question whether or not you have reached ketosis.

After you have brought up your ketone levels, add in some carb-loading days might be an option for you. These carb-loading days shouldn't be used as a cheat day. You need to be careful since any of these high carb days might kick you out of ketosis and then it might take you a week or so to get back into ketosis.

# Chapter 6: Making Keto Work for You

A lot of people choose not to go on a diet because they are afraid that they won't be able to implement it in their lives. The amazing thing about a ketogenic diet is that it is not all that hard to implement, and shouldn't affect your life. To help put everybody's mind at ease about following a keto diet, we are going to look at various ways to make your life easier.

## Budget

Many people will assume that following a keto diet will be expensive, but it doesn't have to be. You will be eating more fat, and this will make you feel fuller than carbs. This means that you won't be eating as much. Since you likely won't need snacks, you'll save money.

Since protein stays about the same, you won't have to buy a bunch of expensive meats. The following are some money-saving tips:

- Keep it simple. You don't have to make fancy meals. The fewer ingredients you need, the more money you will save. If all you have for breakfast is a simple omelet with water, it will cost you about $3.50, if that. A Big Mac is $5.

- Get fresh vegetables when they are in season. The rest of the time, go with frozen.

- Buying a whole chicken and cutting it apart on your own is typically cheaper. You can also use the bones to make your own bone broth.

- Make sure you take notice of deals that your grocery store has, and stock up when things go on sale, especially if you use them a lot.

It's best if you take the time to plan out your shopping list and meals. This will keep you organized. You will make you less likely to buy things that you don't need. Having a shopping list is the best way to keep unnecessary spending at bay.

When you are shopping, here are a few things that you can do to save money:

- Buy block cheese in bulk, and stick to regular cheeses. You can shred your own cheese.

- You can make your own coleslaw, so don't be packaged.

- Purchase simple meats instead of specialty. Cooked meats make a great quick meal but go with things that are less exotic.

- You don't have to worry about kale because it is one of the more expensive greens. You can pick other greens that are cheaper and just as nutritious.

- Avoid nuts as much as you can because they do add up.
- Pick almond meal instead of almond flour. It's cheaper and works just like almond flour. You could also make your own out of almonds.
- Don't buy avocados when not in season.
- Purchase canned or frozen fish instead of fresh, especially if you like salmon.

Get the best quality of food that fits into your budget. Just because everybody tells you that you have to eat organic, doesn't mean you have to listen to them. If something doesn't fit into your budget, don't get it. The most important thing is for you to cook your own meals. They are going to be healthier whether you used organic or not.

When you are choosing meats, go with the cheaper cuts. Never forget to check out those yellow stickers, they normally have a good deal. Cooking meals at home are going to be cheaper than trying to find keto at restaurants.

## Traveling

The most important thing for any diet to be sustainable is being able to eat when not at home. The key to sticking to keto when traveling is to plan things out. Keep the following in mind.

- Be aware of your macros

Before you head out on vacation, you need to make sure that you know your macros. Have them memorized, or have a keto app so that you can track them.

- Evaluate your trip

The next thing you need to do is figure out how long your trip is going to be. If it is only overnight, that will be pretty easy to plan for. A couple of frozen meals, a cooler, and a microwave are all you need. If it is going to be weeklong, that can create some complications. Knowing what you are getting ready to face, though, will help.

After you know the length of the trip and where you are going, you can look at what resources you will have when you arrive. If you can, finding a hotel room with a kitchen is a great idea. Airbnb is a great idea. Finding places that allow you to cook more will improve your flexibility. At the very least, try to find a place that has a full-size fridge and freezer. If you are staying with family or friends, then you have less to worry about.

Knowing how you are traveling is the last thing to worry about. If you are driving, things will be a bit more flexible than if you are on a plane. TSA restrictions will likely prevent you from bringing certain foods because they have to be repacked and weight less than three ounces.

- Food choices

Now you need to think about the foods that you can take with you. Foods that don't have to be refrigerated are great. Things like canned chicken and fish and beef jerky are great. Olives and canned protein shakes are perfect too. All of the regular snack foods like nuts, string cheese, and pepperoni should definitely be packed. If you enjoy eggs, try to hard-boil some.

When it comes to perishables, you will want to buy them once you arrive unless your vacation spot is fairly close to home. You can try packing a cooler with ice to keep things fresh if you want.

Once you arrive, buy some cheese and meats. If you want, you can make all of your meals ahead of time and freeze them before your trip. Pack them up in a cooler and then set them out the morning you want to eat them.

- Restaurants

You can find fast food places and other restaurants that offer low-carb options. You can ask places to wrap your burger in lettuce and leave off the bun. Sticking with steak or fish is great. Avoid fries as the side, as well as rice and beans. Try going for a salad or veggies. If there is a Chipotle nearby, then you can get a bowl without the rice and beans and fill it up with meat, sour cream, cheese, and guacamole.

Travelling doesn't mean if you have to quit eating right. There are a lot of ways to work around these things.

## Keto While Dining Out

There will come a time when you are faced with having to eat out on keto. You don't want to live the rest of your life afraid to go out with your friends and family. Here are some tips to help.

- *Avoid the starch*

Turn down bread, don't order pasta or potatoes, and stay away from rice. Don't allow temptations to touch your plate so order things without starches. The majority of restaurants will allow you to substitute the starchy side for extra vegetables or a salad. If you are in the mood for a burger or sandwich, see if they are willing to wrap it in lettuce instead. If they won't let you make a substitution, then eliminate the item.

If you do get your plate and there is a starch on it, look at your options. If you believe you can keep it on your plate and be tempted not to touch it, then keep it there. If you don't think you can handle it, ask the water to get rid of the starch. If you are at a casual place, you can just throw it out on your own.

- *Add some healthy fats*

Restaurants tend to serve low-fat meals, which makes it hard to feel full without carbs. This can be fixed. Ask them for extra butter that you can add to your veggies or meat. Get a vinaigrette dressing. A seasoned keto dieter will have a small bottle of olive oil with them since restaurants tend to use cheap vegetable oils that have a lot of omega 6 fats.

- ***Pay attention to sauces and condiments***

Sauces like Béarnaise are mainly fats. Ketchup will normally be mostly carbs, and gravies could go either way. If you aren't sure, ask the waiter what's in them so that you don't end up eating hidden carbs. You can also ask to have the sauce on the side so that you can make your own decision on how much.

- ***Be wise on drinks***

The best things to pick are water, sparkling water, coffee, or unsweetened tea. If you want alcohol, pick a dry wine, champagne, or spirits. Spirits should be mixed only with club soda or kept straight.

- ***Dessert***

If you're not hungry, have a cup of coffee or tea while the others have dessert. If you want dessert, go for a cheese plate or berries with whipped cream.

- ***Buffets***

This can become a problem. Create some ground rules for yourself. Stay away from starches and grains and go for the fats, protein, and vegetables. Pick a small plate. You can go back for seconds if you know you are still hungry. Take your time when you eat. Talk with the people you are with and sip on your drink to slow your eating down.

## You're Not a Cook

Maybe you tend to come home late, or you just don't like cooking. You unexpectedly find you don't have the stuff to make something keto. How can you work around these problems?

- ***Have something to drink***

If you are just trying to wait until your next planned meal, have tea or coffee loaded with some healthy fats to help curb your appetite.

- ***Have low-carb snacks***

You don't have to cook. You can make an appetizer plate for your dinner full of healthy, keto snacks.

- ***Have leftovers***

When do cook, make enough so that you can have leftovers on those days when don't want to cook.

- ***Use a slow cooker***

This is perfect if you do work late. You can prep this in the morning, and it will be ready for you when you get home.

## Holidays

Holidays are the worst for diets, but if you don't want to mess up your new good habit, a little planning can go a long way. The most important thing is not to be the annoying dieter who tries to keep others from eating what they want. Keep yourself composed. You eat what you want to eat, and they can have what they want.

If you are visiting family and you want to find out what is normally in certain dishes that you didn't fix, there's an app for that. This will help you to make smart decisions. If you tend to find yourself coveting that cake on the dessert table, make sure you volunteer to take the dessert. Make a dessert or two that you know that you can have without any fear.

It also helps to try to avoid debating with others. You are seeing family you likely don't see very often, and they may give you a hard time for your new eating style. On the other hand, you may feel like bragging. Its best, though, not to engage. You're not there to fix the way your family eats. Look out for yourself.

The last thing, it is the holidays, and if you slip, it is not the end of the world. If you don't want to break your mom or grandma's heart by turning down their signature dish, then eat some of it. Get a little bit and enjoy it. You can have a few of the goodies, just know your limits and don't go hog wild. Enjoy yourself and listen to your body. You don't have to be super strict all the time. Just make sure you don't let yourself fall completely off the wagon.

# Chapter 7: What You Should and Shouldn't Eat

You know the basics of a ketogenic diet, and you know, pretty much, what you should and shouldn't do. Now is the time to find out exactly what foods you can and can't eat while on a ketogenic diet.

## What You Shouldn't Eat

We'll start with everything that you need to cut out of your diet, or at least greatly reduced.

- Sugar – this is the biggest no-no. You have to get rid of vitamin water, sports drinks, fruit juices, and soft drinks. Also:
    - Breakfast cereals
    - Frozen treats
    - Donuts
    - Chocolate bars
    - Cookies
    - Cakes
    - Candy
    - Sweets
- Beer – this is basically liquid bread.
- Fruit
- Margarine – you want to use real butter, not the fake butter.
- Pre-packaged low-carb foods – make sure you read the label before you buy these. Even Atkins products aren't all low-carb.
- Starch:
    - Muesli
    - Porridge
    - Potato chips
    - French fries

- Sweet potatoes
- Potatoes
- Rice
- Pasta
- Bread
- Lentils
- Beans

## Foods You Should Eat

Now that you know what you need to avoid, let's look at everything that you get to enjoy while on a ketogenic diet.

- Dark chocolate – aim for finding chocolate that has a cocoa amount of more than 70%. 85% is the ideal cocoa amount.
- Alcohol – if you must have alcohol, try dry wine, vodka, brandy, whiskey, and anything that doesn't have sugar added.
- Water – this is a must-have.
- Coffee – make sure you don't add anything except for butter or coconut oil.
- Tea – any tea you would like, just don't add sugar.
- Bone broth – this can help add electrolytes and nutrients.
- Berries – these are good in moderation. These include raspberries, blackberries, strawberries, and blueberries.
- High-fat dairy – the more fat, the better. Butter is the best, and high-fat cheeses are good. High-fat yogurts should be consumed in moderation. Regular milk has too much sugar, so avoid it.
- Nuts – you can have these in moderation. The best are macadamia, Brazil, and pecans.
- Above ground vegetables – pick vegetables that are grown above the ground, especially green vegetables. The best are:
    - Cauliflower
    - Cabbage
    - Avocado

- Broccoli
- Zucchini
- Spinach
- Asparagus
- Kale
- Green beans
- Brussels sprouts

- Seafood and fish – these are all great options, especially salmon, which is high in fat.

- Eggs – these are great because you can fix them in all different ways.

- High-fat sauces – a lot of the fat you eat should come from natural sources like eggs, fish, and meat, but you can also use fats to cook, such as coconut oil and butter.

- Meats – all unprocessed meats are low in carbs and great for keto. The best are grass-fed and organic meats. You have to remember that you're supposed to eat high in fats and not proteins, so don't go crazy. Watch out for processed meats like meatballs, sausages, and cold cuts. They sometimes have added carbs.

# Chapter 8: Is It Right for You

While the keto diet is a great and effective tool for weight loss, it may not be the right diet for you. Chances are, before reading this book, you had heard about the keto diet and decided that it was just another fad that won't last, but it has been followed for over 100 years. You are already aware of all the health benefits that the diet brings, and all of this is due to ketosis. But, it is this ketone adaptation that can cause some safety problems that you need to keep in mind. This is why I have provided you with this chapter because it may not be a good idea for everybody. The following are some situations where a ketogenic diet may be dangerous. While you may still be able to follow it, you will want to exercise caution and do so under a doctor's supervision.

## Pregnant or Nursing

There aren't a lot of studies done on the effects of a keto diet on a pregnant woman. Some studies, though, have found that some side effects could include weight loss, anemia, nutrient deficiency, hormonal changes, dehydration, inadequate growth in the fetus, and constipation.

Prolong ketosis while pregnant could end up causing developmental problems for the baby that can end up affecting the development of their brain and increases the risk of defects, such as spina bifida. Due to the problems that it could cause for the baby, doctors do not recommend this diet for pregnant women.

Much like with a pregnant woman, there aren't too many studies about what keto can do to a nursing woman. Most women who are nursing or pregnant often need more protein and fiber than other women. The increased fiber helps to support the development and growth of the fetus, helps with their digestion, and provides both mom and baby with the vitamins and minerals they need.

Since we don't know for certain the exact results of a ketogenic diet on nursing women, it is best to follow a moderate carb intake that is safe for the mother and the baby.

## Medication-Caused Hypoglycemia

The most common hypoglycemia-causing medications are:

- Insulin

- Sulphonylureas, such as glibenclamide, tolbutamide, gliclazide, glipizide, and glimepiride.

- Glinides, such as nateglinide or repaglinide.

All of these medications are made to help increase insulin in the body. This will then lower a person's blood sugar levels. If you are following a ketogenic diet while on these medications, it could increase your odds of developing hypoglycemia. It is important that you speak your doctor so that both of you can work together to prevent you from developing hypoglycemia before you start keto.

Making sure that you take regular blood glucose tests will give you the ability to spot and avoid developing hypoglycemia. You will have to perform tests more often than normal while your body works to adjust to the change of carbohydrate intake.

## Diabetes or Blood Sugar Problems

There are plenty of people who suffer from diabetes or blood sugar problems that can follow a keto diet without any problems. There are some, however, who try to follow a keto diet and will suffer from low blood sugar when they first start. This can turn out to be dangerous if you are unable to stabilize your blood sugar while on diabetes medications.

There is a lot of evidence that shows that diabetes can be slowed or prevents through a healthy diet and exercise. To be on the safe side, people who have a history of hypoglycemia, prediabetes, or diabetes should consult with their doctor before they begin a ketogenic diet.

Changes in your diet and weight loss could mean that you need to change your diabetes medication dosage. Only your doctor can make these. You should never change your medication without talking with your doctor first.

## On Other Medications

The majority of medications won't cause a significant risk, but you should still to do some research and speak with your doctor to make sure there won't be any problems. Your doctor will know if they need to change the dosage. Blood pressure medications could end up needing to be regulated more by your physician because a keto diet could cause your blood pressure to drop too low.

## Underweight or Nutrient Deficient

The ketogenic diet is meant as a way to lose weight, and weight loss tends to happen quickly. If you are currently underweight, have vitamin or mineral deficiencies due to not eating right, or have suffered from past eating disorders, this is not the right diet for you. If your BMI is in the underweight range and you want to follow a keto diet to improve your blood sugar levels, and you don't want to lose weight, please talk to your doctor to help you to modify the diet to ensure that your weight isn't affected.

If you tend to lose weight easily, a diet with more complex carbs along with plenty of healthy fats and proteins is the best thing. If you have ever undergone gastric bypass surgery, the ketogenic diet may be dangerous because of the risk of nutrient deficiencies that can happen from not consuming enough calories.

## Children

While there have been many children suffering from epileptic seizures who have been treated with a ketogenic diet, they were under medical supervision. There are many different things that you need to remember before starting a ketogenic diet for a child is to make sure that the macronutrients are balanced and appropriate for them. You absolutely must speak with a doctor or dietitian before you allow your child to start a keto diet.

## Kidney Disease or Stones

The keto diet has the ability to cause kidney stones. If you already have a history of kidney disease, it probably isn't worth it to try and follow a ketogenic diet. If you have a history of any type of kidney disease, you have to talk with your doctor before you start this type of diet. Your doctor will need to keep an eye on your creatinine/calcium ratio to make sure that you aren't suffering from complications like nephrolithiasis, which is very dangerous calcium levels in your kidneys.

## Gallstones or Gall Bladder Removal

People who suffer from gallstones are often told to stay away from fat, but that isn't necessarily the case anymore. The NHS says that a low-fat diet can cause gallstone growth. If you already suffer from gallstones, consuming more fat could cause more pain. If you are interested in a ketogenic diet, you may want to slowly start the diet or wait until your gallstones have been removed.

A study in 2014 found that high-fat diets could prevent the formation of gallstones, which could be another long-term benefit of this diet. The gall bladder has bile in it that will help your body to break down fats so it may not seem like a smart idea to follow a high-fat diet like a ketogenic diet. There are plenty of people, though, that have had their gall bladder removed that have successfully followed the diet without any adverse effects.

## Enzyme Deficiency or Defect

These are both very rare problems, but there are two big contraindications of the ketogenic diet called pyruvate carboxylase and porphyria deficiency. These are both caused by issues with the production of lipid and heme metabolism. Heme is part of the hemoglobin that carries oxygen out of the lungs and into other areas of your body.

People who suffer from these disorders will also suffer from deficiencies with some enzymes that make it hard for them to metabolize large amounts of fatty acids. They are then transported to the cell's mitochondria to make energy. If you follow this type of diet and suffer from these deficiencies or other types of beta oxidations defects, it can create dangerous complications like irregular heartbeats, nervous system deterioration, and mental changes.

Free fatty acids will build up, but the body won't be able to sue them for energy, and this is why it becomes dangerous. People who have pyruvate carboxylase and porphyria deficiency need a good supply of glucose to provide their organs with energy. If there is no glucose present because of this diet, some life-threatening problems can occur. This is known as a catabolic crisis. To avoid these problems, if you have a family history of mitochondrial disorders or you think you may have these conditions, you need to have a doctor test you before even thinking about starting a ketogenic diet.

# Chapter 9: Lose 21 Pounds in 21 Days

Now has come the time for your kick-start to your ketogenic diet. We will look at each week individually as well as the meal prep journey that you will need to take. The recipes for these first 21-days will also be in this chapter as well. You can continue to use the recipes after the initial 21-day diet.

It may look as if there are not enough meals here for an entire week, but the idea here is to make meal prep easy and simple. This means that you won't have to cook for every single meal, making it easier to stick with the diet. While you will be eating the same meals a few times a week, you have the ability to alternate the days you eat them so that you don't have to eat the same things two days in a row. This will keep things from getting boring.

Each meal has a standard serving size. However, you are allowed to adjust this serving to be more or less depending on what you daily macro needs are.

There is no set menu with this; you can pick and choose what you want to have for breakfast, lunch, and dinner every day. The snacks are there if you need them. You don't have to eat a snack if you don't feel like you need one. Having them on hand is always good though. Just as an example, you could have:

- Monday
    - Roasted Avocado and Egg – Breakfast
    - Cesar Salad – Lunch
    - Burrito Bowl – Dinner
    - Buttercream Fat Bomb – Dessert
- Tuesday
    - Bacon, Eggs, and Tomatoes – Breakfast
    - Fresh Tomato and Sardine Salad – Lunch
    - Deviled Egg – Snack
    - Salami Basil Pizza – Dinner

Ultimately, what you eat each day is up to you.

## Week One

**Breakfast:**

Bacon, Eggs, and Tomatoes

Roasted Avocado and Egg

**Lunch:**

Fresh Tomato and Sardine Salad

Cesar Salad

**Dinner:**

Burrito Bowls

Thai Shrimp Curry Noodles

Salami Basil Pizza

**Snacks:**

Bacon Deviled Eggs

Buttercream Fat Bombs

Pistachio Almond Fat Bombs

Like what you're reading? Want to hear this as an audio book? Click here to get this book for FREE when you join Audible!!

https://adbl.co/2YmbdC8

# Roasted Avocado and Egg

This dish isn't the best dish to try and cook in advance. However, all of the ingredients can be prepped at the start of the week, so that you will only have to put it together, which takes about three minutes, and then cook it for 15 minutes.

The toppings and measurements for them are optional, so the nutritional information is only for the egg and avocado. One standard serving has 465 calories, 3 g net carbs, 39 g fat, and 17 g protein.

**What you need:**

Favorite cheese

Pepper

Salt

Cilantro

Chopped chives

Sliced ham

Eggs, 2

Avocado, 1

**What you do:**

- Start by placing your oven at 40 and prepare a glass pan.
- Slice the avocado in half and take out the pit. Scrape out a small amount of flesh to make the hole big enough for an egg.
- Put the avocado halves in the pan and crack an egg into the middle of each, and then add on your toppings of choice.
- Let your avocados bake for 15 minutes, or until the yolk is set to your desired consistency. Top with cilantro and chives if you want.

# Bacon, Eggs, and Tomatoes

The bacon and tomatoes can be cooked ahead of time. They can be reheated as you cook your eggs. This recipe makes only one serving and contains 380 calories, 7 g net carbs, 27 g fat, 21 g protein.

**What you need:**

Pepper

Salt

Roma tomatoes, 2

Bacon fat, 2 tsp.

Bacon, 2 strips

Eggs, 2

**What you do:**

- On the day that you prep your meals, set your oven to 400. Place aluminum foil on a baking sheet and top with a wire cooling rack. Assemble another pan, a small glass one.

- Put the bacon strips on the cooling rack and back for 15 to 20 minutes until crispy. Pour the extra fat into a glass jar so that you can use it later.

- At the same time as you cook your bacon, roast your tomatoes in the glass pan. First, you need to wash and dry the tomatoes and let them roast for 25 to 30 minutes.

- Keep the bacon and tomatoes stored in the fridge until the morning that you plan on having this for breakfast. You can reheat them in the microwave or skillet and add some pepper and salt to the tomatoes.

- Cook your eggs the morning of in any fashion that you desire using some of the reserved bacon fat. Season and serve alongside the tomatoes and bacon.

# Cesar Salad

You will need mason jars for this. They allow you to assemble the salads on your prep day and you won't have to worry about the lettuce becoming soggy. One serving contains 626 calories, 50 g fat, 7 g net carbs, and 35 g protein.

**What you need:**

Pepper

Salt

Onion powder

Garlic powder

Primal Kitchen's Cesar dressing, 2 tbsp.

Parmesan cheese, 4 tbsp.

Bone-in chicken thighs, 2

Romaine lettuce, 2 servings

**What you do:**

- All of this will be done on your prep day. The only thing you have to do on the day that you eat it is to shake the salad in the jar and enjoy.
- Start by placing your oven on 375. In a glass pan, place the chicken thighs in it and top with some seasonings. Allow them to roast for 25 to 35 minutes or until they are fully cooked and it reaches 165.
- If you didn't by pre-washed and torn lettuce, you would need to wash, tear, and dry your lettuce.
- Once the chicken is cooked and cooled, debone and slice it up, keeping the skin on.
- Divide the ingredients into two portions.
- Put the dressing at the bottom of two quart-sized mason jars, add in the cheese, the chicken, and then top with the lettuce. This order is very important because it will keep your lettuce crunchy.

# Tomato and Sardine Salad

This recipe makes three servings and has 419 calories, 7 g net carbs, 31 g fat, and 27 g protein.

**What you need:**

Apple cider vinegar, 1 tbsp.

Dijon mustard, 2 tsp.

Celery, 2 ribs

Olive oil, 1 tbsp.

Blue cheese, .25 c

Chopped walnuts, .33 c

Heirloom tomatoes, 1.5 lbs.

Herbes de Provence

Salt

Drained capers, 2 tbsp.

Canned sardines, boneless and skinless in olive oil, 3 cans

**What you do:**

- To prep, the sardines, turn your broil on and open up the cans. Top them with a tablespoon of capers, herbs de Provence, and salt.
- Cook in the oven until they are hot. The oil should be bubbling. This will take three to five minutes.
- Wash and slice the tomatoes into bite-sized pieces.
- Slice the celery. Toast the walnuts in a pan until fragrant. The nuts can burn quickly, so make sure you watch them. This will take around a minute.
- Add the seasonings, olive oil, mustard, and vinegar in a bowl and whisk together.
- Layer the salad in quart-sized mason jars. Place the vinaigrette on the bottom then add the walnuts, blue cheese, celery, tomatoes, and sardines.
- You can serve it in the jar or pour it out in a plate when you are ready to eat.

# Thai Shrimp Curry Noodles

The shrimp can be replaced with chicken if you have an allergy or if you don't like shrimp. This makes four servings, and one serving has 199 calories, 10 g net carbs, 12 g fat, and 12 g protein.

**What you need:**

Butternut squash "noodles" or spaghetti squash, 2 c

Salt, 2 tsp.

Thai red curry paste, 1 tbsp.

Sliced mushrooms, 8 oz.

Diced onion, 1 medium

Canned full-fat coconut milk, .5 c

Deveined large shrimp with tails removed, 10 oz.

**What you do:**

- If using spaghetti squash, place the whole squash in a 9 x 13 pan with a cup or so of water. Roast at 375 for a few hours, or until you can pierce it easily with a knife. Once it is cooled, slice in half to remove the seeds, and then use a fork to flake the meat out of the inside. It will look like noodles.

- If using butternut squash, you can spiralize your own noodles, or you can buy pre-spiralized butternut squash noodles in the produce department. Depending on where you shop, you may have a hard time finding pre-spiralized. Toss them in olive oil and salt, and the roast them at 375 for around 15 to 20 minutes, or until tender.

- Place the mushrooms and onions in a pot with the olive oil and sauté for around ten minutes.

- Mix in the salt, red curry paste, and coconut milk. Bring everything up to a simmer.

- Once it is simmering, add in the shrimp, cover the pot, and allow it to cook until the shrimp turn pink about ten minutes.

- Serve the mixture over your chosen noodles. Only use half of a cup of butternut squash noodles or one cup of spaghetti squash.

# Burrito Bowls

This recipe makes four servings. One standard serving has 380 calories, 13 g net carbs, 24 g fat, and 22 g protein.

**What you need:**

Shredded cheddar cheese, .5 c

Sour cream, .5 c

Guacamole, 1.5 c

Cilantro, .33 c

Diced tomatoes, 2

Lettuce, 340 grams

Salt, 2 tsp.

Olive oil, 2 tbsp.

Cauliflower rice, 3 c

Water, 1 c

Chili powder, 1 tsp.

Cumin, .5 tsp.

Minced garlic, 3 cloves

Diced onion, 1

Paprika, .5 tsp.

Sea salt, 3 tsp.

Juice and zest of a lime

Beef tips, .5 lb.

**What you do:**

- In a pressure cooker, add the beef tips, water, paprika, cumin, chili powder, garlic, onion, salt, and lime. Place the pressure cooker on high pressure and let it cook for 20 minutes. Allow all of the pressure to release naturally, or wait ten minutes before using the manual pressure release.

- Cauliflower rice can be found the frozen food aisle and the produce department. You can also rice your own if you want. Place the cauliflower on a parchment lined baking sheet, toss with some oil and two teaspoons of salt, and pat it down so that it is flat. Roast for 15 minutes at 400. Stir, and then cook for another five minutes.

- To serve everything, place the rice and the meat in a bowl and then top everything with the cold ingredients.

# Salami Basil Pizza

This recipe makes four servings. One standard serving has 409 calories, 8 g net carbs, 30 g fat, and 27 g protein.

**What you need:**

Olive oil, 1 tbsp.

Pepper, .25 tsp.

Salt, .5 tsp.

Sliced basil, 10 leaves

Chopped Hormel Natural Choice salami, 4 sliced

Shredded mozzarella, 3 c

Victoria's marinara sauce, .5 c

Italian seasoning, 1 tsp.

Egg, 1

Parmesan or mozzarella cheese, .5 c

Cauliflower rice, 6 c

**What you do:**

- Place your oven to 400. Line a baking sheet with parchment paper.
- Pour the cauliflower rice on the baking sheet and allow it to cook for 15 minutes.
- Once the cauliflower has cooled for about five minutes, place it on some cheesecloth. Form it into a ball in the middle of the cloth and squeeze out the liquid. Try to squeeze out as much liquid as you can. The crust will hold up better the dryer you can make the cauliflower.
- Turn the oven up to 450.
- Mix together the cauliflower, mozzarella or parmesan, seasonings, and egg.

- Line a baking sheet with parchment paper. Form four round mini pizza crusts on the pan. Brush the tops of the cuts with olive oil.

- Allow it to bake for 15 minutes. With a spatula, carefully flip them over and let them cook for five more minutes.

- At this point, you can allow them to cool completely and store them in a plastic bag in the fridge for up to five days, or you can freeze them for a month.

- Once you are ready to make your pizzas. Allow the crusts to unthaw completely. Top them with the sauce, cheese, salami, and basil. Bake them at 400 until the cheese is golden and bubbly.

## Buttercream Fat Bombs

This recipe makes around a dozen fat bombs if you use a traditional cookie scoop, which is about four teaspoons. One standard fat bomb has 138 calories, 5 g net carbs, 14 g fat, and 2 g protein.

**What you need:**

Lily's dark chocolate, 8 oz.

Vanilla extract, 1 tsp.

Fine salt, .25 tsp.

Sugar-free Truvia, .33 c

Full-fat cream cheese, room temp, .5 c

Grass-fed butter, room temp, .5 c

**What you do:**

- Mix together the vanilla, salt, sweetener, cream cheese, and butter until fully combined. You want to make sure that everything is well mixed; otherwise, you could end up with clumps of salt and vanilla.

- Chill for at least two hours, and then scoop out with a small cookie scoop. Place on a pan and allow to chill for another hour.

- Melt the chocolate, and then dip the fat bombs into it. Chill until set, about two hours.

# Pistachio Almond Fat Bombs

This recipe makes 20 servings. One serving has 202 calories, 1.8 g net carbs, 21 g fat, and 1.7 g protein.

**What you need:**

Coconut butter, .5 c

Almond butter, .5 c

Chopped pistachios, 3 tbsp.

Ground cinnamon, .5 tsp.

Salt, .25 tsp.

Ground nutmeg, .25 tsp.

Ground cardamom, .25 tsp.

Pepper, .25 tsp.

Vanilla, 1 tsp.

Sugar-free Truvia, .25 c

Softened butter, 2 tbsp.

Chilled full-fat coconut milk, .25 c

Melted cacao butter, .25 c

Firm coconut oil, .25 c

**What you do:**

- Line a 9-inch square dish with parchment paper.

- Place all of the ingredients in a blender, except for the pistachios and cacao butter. Blend everything together on high until the ingredients are fully combined and airy.

- Pour the cacao butter in and continue to blend until well incorporated.

- Pour into the pan and sprinkle the top with the pistachios. Chill overnight.

- Slice into 20 squares.

## Bacon Deviled Eggs

This makes 12 deviled eggs. Two deviled egg has 193 calories, 0 g net carbs, 17 g fat, and 8 g protein.

**What you need:**

Mayonnaise, .25 c

Cooked bacon, 3 slices

Eggs, 6

Salt

Sliced green onions, 1 stalk

Garlic and onion powder, to taste

Dijon mustard, 1 tsp.

**What you do:**

- Place the eggs in water and bring to a boil. Allow them to boil for 15 minutes and then place them in cold water. Allow them to cool completely and then peel the eggs.

- Slice them in half and remove the yolks to a bowl. Smash the yolks with a fork until they are fine.

- Stir in the seasonings, Dijon, and mayonnaise.

- Scoop the mixture into the egg whites and top with the bacon and green onions.

## Week Two

While having a lot of meal choices is nice, every additional recipe you have to cook is going to take up more of your time. In week two you will find even more recipes, but if you want to limit your prep and planning, you can limit the recipes to around two per meal type. However, it is nice to have more meal options when you start a keto diet because they will likely help to stave off your cravings.

## Breakfast:

Bulletproof Coffee

Breakfast Cheese Tacos

Chocolate Shake

## Lunch:

Turnip Green Wraps

Bacon Cheeseburger

Cobb Salad

## Dinner:

Lemon Butter Chicken with Mac and Cheese

Egg Roll Bowls

Jalapeno Popper Casserole

## Snacks:

Red Hot Cauliflower Bites

Raspberry Almond Bark

Lemon Cheesecake Fat Bombs

Chocolate Chip Cookie Dough Fat Bombs

# Chocolate Shake

This is great for those who find themselves not as hungry in the morning. It makes one serving that contains 256 calories, 8 g net carbs, 18 g fat, and 10 g protein.

### What you need:

Chocolate exogenous ketones, 1 scoop

Cocoa powder, 2 tbsp.

Unsweetened full-fat yogurt, 3 tbsp.

Tahini paste, .5 tbsp.

Stevia drops, 10

Water, .75 c

Egg yolks, 2

### What you do:

- Place all of the ingredients in a blender and pulse until everything is blended.

# Cheesy Breakfast Tacos

This makes one serving as has 253 calories, 57 g fat, and 33 g protein.

### What you need:

Shredded cheddar cheese, 3 oz.

Egg, 1

Cilantro, 2 sprigs

Salt

Diced tomato, 2 tbsp.

Arugula, .25 c

Grass-fed butter, 1 tsp.

Bacon, 2 slices

**What you do:**

- On the day that you prep your meals, back your bacon in the oven at 400 for about 15 minutes. Measure out all of the ingredients that you need so that it is easier to assemble on the day you make this.

- On the day you want to have the tacos, warm the bacon in the microwave as you prep everything else.

- Warm a skillet and add the butter. Melt, and then sprinkle in the cheese to make a round taco shell. Once the cheese has melted as is bubbling, crack an egg on top and sprinkle with salt.

- Once the egg turn opaque and cheese has started to brown, cover with a lid and turn down to low. Allow to cook for another two minutes.

- Carefully take the taco out of the pan and place it on a cutting board. With two bowls or cups, use them to form the cheese into the shape of a shell. Let it cool until hard.

- Add in the cilantro, tomato, arugula, and bacon.

## Bulletproof Coffee

One standard serving has 474 calories, 3 g net carbs, 45.6 g fat, and 15 g protein.

**What you need:**

Pumpkin pie spice, .5 tsp. (optional)

Sugar-free Swerve, 1 tsp.

Collagen, 1 tbsp.

Full-fat coconut milk, 2 tbsp.

Ghee, 1 tbsp.

3 egg yolks

MCT oil, 1 tbsp.

Hot coffee, 8 oz.

**What you do:**

- Place everything in a blender and mix until frothy and smooth.

## Cobb Salad

You can't completely make this in advance, you can still prep the majority of the ingredients to save time later in the week. This recipe is one serving and has 901 calories, 8 g net carbs, 50 g fat, and 50 g protein.

**What you need:**

Tessemae's Lemon Garlic salad dressing, 2 tbsp.

Shredded cheddar cheese, .25 c

Sliced hardboiled egg

Sliced avocado, .5

Chopped cooked bacon, 1 slice

Sliced cooked chicken thigh

Chopped and washed romaine lettuce, 4 c

**What you do:**

- Place all of the ingredients in a bowl and toss with the salad dressing.

# Bacon Cheeseburger

This recipe makes one burger and has 485 calories, 9 g net carbs, 65 g fat, and 50 g protein.

**What you need:**

Iceberg lettuce, several large leaves

Sliced tomato, .5

Mayonnaise, 1 tbsp.

Cheddar cheese, 1 slice

Bacon, 2 slices

Salt, .5 tsp.

Pepper

Garlic powder, .25 tsp.

Onion powder, .25 tsp.

Ground beef, .33 lb.

**What you do:**

- Cook the bacon to your desired doneness. Set aside, but make sure you keep the bacon grease. Mix together the pepper, salt, onion powder, garlic powder, and the ground beef as the bacon cooks. Form the beef into a patty.

- Turn up the heat on the pan with the bacon grease. You can grill the burger if you would like. Cook for four minutes on each side. When you are cooking the second side, you can place the cheese slice on the burger to let it melt.

- Get the veggies prepped as your burger cooks. Pat the lettuce dry.

- To assemble the burgers, place one or two lettuce leaves on a plate and spread on the mayonnaise. Add on the burger and then the bacon. Finally, top with a couple more lettuce leaves.

# Turnip Green Wraps

This makes one wrap and has 594 calories, 7 g net carbs, 55 g fat, and 34 g protein.

**What you need:**

Keto mayonnaise, 1 tbsp.

Sliced turkey or chicken, 4 oz.

Sliced avocado, .5

Cooked bacon, 2 slices

Sliced Roma tomato, 1

Large, washed, turnip green leaves, 2

**What you do:**

- Remove the excess tough stem from the base of the turnip greens. You want to leave most of the stem on the turnip green.
- Smear the mayonnaise on the leaves and layer on the meat, bacon, avocado, and tomato.
- Wrap up and enjoy.

# Jalapeno Popper Casserole

This whole thing can easily be made ahead of time and store either in the freezer or the fridge until you want to enjoy it. This makes three servings, and each serving has 482 calories, 3 g net carbs, 38 g fat, and 26 g protein

**What you need:**

Pepper, .25 tsp.

Onion powder, .75 tsp.

Sea salt, .5 tsp. + .5 tsp.

Minced garlic, 2 cloves

Monterey jack cheese, .25 c

Cheddar cheese, .25 c

Heavy cream, 2 tbsp.

Full-fat cream cheese, 3 oz.

Cooked and crumbled bacon, 3 slices

Jalapeno peppers, 3

Boneless and skinless chicken thighs, 12 oz.

**What you do:**

- Start by setting your oven to 400 and grease a 9-inch square pan.

- Chop the chicken thighs into one-inch cubes. Heat up an oiled pan and add in the chicken. Season with pepper and half of the salt.

- As the chicken is cooking, prep the jalapenos by removing their seeds. Mince two of the jalapenos up and slice the third into rounds.

- Once the chicken has cooked completely, stir in the cream cheese and heavy cream. Mix until well combined.

- Stir in the minced jalapeno, three quarters of the crumbled bacon, the Monterey jack cheese, and half of the cheddar. Stir until the cheese has melted and is combined into the other ingredients. Add in the rest of the salt, onion, and garlic. Stir until combined and set it off the heat.

- Pour the mixture into the prepared pan. Top everything with the remaining cheddar, sliced jalapenos, and bacon.

- Bake the dish for ten minutes and then flip the oven up to broiler. Allow it to cook for two more minutes until the cheese begins to turn golden and bubble.

## Egg Roll Bowls

This recipe makes four servings, and each has 453 calories, 7 g net carbs, 30 g fat, and 33 g protein.

**What you need:**

Sesame seeds, 2 tbsp.

Salt, 2 tsp.

Coconut aminos, 3 tbsp.

Rice vinegar, 1 tbsp.

Ground ginger, 5 tsp.

Coleslaw mix, 14 oz.

Red chili flakes, 1 tsp.

Ground beef, .5 lb.

Ground pork, .5 lb.

Sliced green onions, 4 stalks

Minced garlic, 4 cloves

Diced onion, 1 med

Sesame oil, 2 tbsp.

**What you do:**

- Heat up a pan and add in the sesame oil, white portion of the green onions, garlic, and onion. Sauté everything until the garlic is fragrant and the onions have turned translucent.
- Add in the salt, ginger, red pepper flakes, beef, and pork. Cook everything until the meat is fully cooked.
- Stir in the rice vinegar, coconut aminos, and coleslaw mix. Allow it to cook until the coleslaw has become tender.
- Serve topped with the green part of the green onions and sesame seeds.

## Lemon Butter Chicken

This can be fully fixed ahead of time and stored in the fridge for a week, or the freezer for a month. This makes two servings, and a single serving has 713 calories, 6 g net carbs, 55 g fat, and 47 g protein.

**What you need:**

Sea salt, 1 tsp.

Baby spinach, 1 c

Thyme, .25 tsp.

Minced garlic, 3 cloves

Lemon juice, 2 tbsp.

Lemon zest, 1 tsp.

Paprika, 1 tsp.

Grass-fed butter, 2 tbsp.

Parmesan cheese, 2 tbsp.

Chicken broth, 5 c

Heavy cream, .25 c

Bone-in with skin chicken thighs, 2

**What you do:**

- Start by placing your oven to 400.
- Rub your chicken with paprika and sea salt. Heat a cast iron skillet and add in a tablespoon of butter. Place the chicken in the pan sear for three minutes on both sides.
- Remove the chicken and set aside.
- Add the rest of the butter and garlic. Cook until fragrant.
- Stir in the lemon zest, juice, thyme, and chicken broth. Bring up to a boil and allow it to thicken for about seven minutes.
- Turn the heat down and stir in the heavy cream and parmesan. Allow it to cook for a few more minutes.
- Mix in the spinach, and cook until the sauce thickens and the spinach has wilted. Place the chicken back in the pan.
- Place the chicken in the oven and let it cook for 25 minutes, or until it reaches 165.

# Mac and Cheese

This makes four servings, and each contains 283 calories, 6 g net carbs, 23 g fat, and 11 g protein.

**What you need:**

Salt, 2 tsp.

Pepper, .25 tsp.

Turmeric, .5 tsp.

Garlic powder, .5 tsp.

Onion powder, .5 tsp.

Dijon mustard, .5 tsp.

Heavy cream, .5 c

Full-fat cream cheese, cubed, 4 oz.

Sharp shredded cheddar cheese, 4 oz.

Microwave steam bag cauliflower florets, 1 lb.

**What you do:**

- Cook the cauliflower according to the directions on the package.
- Add the heavy cream to a pan and let it come to a simmer. Add in the cream cheese and stir until it is melted. Add in two-thirds of the cheddar and mix until melted.
- Add in all of the seasonings and mix completely. Stir in the cauliflower until coated.
- Sprinkle with the rest of the cheese and stir until combined.

# Chocolate Chip Cookie Dough Fat Bombs

This makes 39 fat bombs, and each fat bomb contains 56 calories, .5 g net carbs, 5.5 g fat, and 1 g protein.

**What you need:**

Salt, .25 tsp.

Vanilla, 1 tsp.

Lily's dark chocolate chips, .25 c

Almond butter, .5 c

Sugar-free Truvia, 3 tbsp.

Perfect keto powdered MCT oil, 6 scoops

Full-fat softened cream cheese, 6 tbsp.

Grass-fed butter, 6 tbsp.

**What you do:**

- Blend together the butter and cream cheese in a blender. Mix in the salt, vanilla, almond butter, sweetener, and MCT powder until completely combined.
- Fold in the chocolate chips.
- Freeze for 10 to 15 minutes.
- Scoop the mixture out on wax paper with a small cookie scoop.
- Place back in the freezer until set and place them in a container and keep in the freezer.

# Lemon Cheesecake Fat Bombs

This makes 12 servings, and each contains 101 calories, .3 g net carbs, 11 g fat, and .6 g protein.

**What you need:**

Salt

Sugar-free Truvia, 2-4 tbsp.

Lemon zest, 1 tbsp.

Lemon juice, 2 tsp.

Melted coconut oil, .25 c

Softened grass-fed butter, .25 c

Softened full-fat cream cheese, 4 oz.

**What you do:**

- Combine the butter, and cream cheese with an electric mixer until airy and sooth.
- Add in the oil, lemon juice, lemon zest, salt, and sweetener. Combine everything together well with a hand mixer.
- Pour into 12 silicone molds or a glass pan.
- Freeze for four to eight hours, top with extra zest if you want. If you use a glass pan, cut them into 12 squares.
- These should be kept in the fridge or the freezer.

# Raspberry Almond Bark

This will make 16 servings, and one serving contains 186 calories, 4.5 g net carbs, 15 g fat, and 4.4 g protein.

**What you need:**

Salt, .25 tsp.

Stevia, .5 tsp.

Cocoa powder, 2 tbsp.

Frozen raspberries, .5 c

Chopped and toasted walnuts, 40 grams

Chopped and toasted almonds, 40 grams

Softened coconut butter, 1 c

Almond butter, 1 c

**What you do:**

- Place parchment into a 9 x 13 pan.
- Using a blender, mix together the almond and coconut butter. Once it is combined, add in the cocoa powder, salt, and stevia.
- In the pan, add the chocolate mixture, and then top it with nuts.
- Place the frozen raspberries in the microwave for a minute so that they become mushy. Scatter over top of the chocolate along with the almonds and walnuts.
- Place the bark in the freezer for no less than an hour. Break into 16 equal size pieces of bark and keep stored in the freezer.

## Red Hot Cauliflower Bites

This makes two servings, and each serving contains 222 calories, 5 g net carbs, 21 g fat, and 4 g protein.

**What you need:**

Blue cheese dressing, 4 tbsp.

Sea salt, 1 tsp.

Melted grass-fed butter, 1 tbsp.

Garlic powder, 1 tsp.

Hot sauce, .33 c

Cauliflower florets, 1 head or 3 c

**What you do:**

- Set your oven to 400. Place parchment on a baking sheet.
- Mix together the sea salt, garlic powder, hot sauce, and melted butter. Add in the cauliflower and toss it all together.
- Place on the baking sheet and roast for 18 to 20 minutes.
- Serve with blue cheese or ranch dressing.

## Week Three

Congratulations on making it through the first two weeks. By now, you have probably figured out which dishes you like the best and which ones you will incorporate into your regular diet. You will also probably know how many different meals you are comfortable with meal prepping for the week.

This is your third and final week. After this, you can come up with your own menu by combining the recipes from these three weeks, and the other recipes that you will find in the rest of the book. You will find what works best for you.

## Breakfast:

Cream Cheese Danish

Hash Browns, Bacon, and Eggs

Chai Tea Latte

## Lunch:

Broccoli Cheddar Soup

Chicken Salad

Lasagna Bowls

## Dinner:

Beef Stroganoff Meatballs with Noodles

Butter Salmon with Capers and Zucchini Gratin

Chicken Cordon Bleu Casserole

**Snacks:**
Peppermint Mocha Drops

Mocha Bonbons

Broccoli Cheddar Tots

## Chai Tea Latte

You can prepare a large batch of the spice mixture to make things faster when you fix this. One standard serving has 254 calories, 8 g net carbs, 68 g fat, and 5 g protein.

**What you need:**

Latte

Chair blend, 1 tsp.

Black tea, 2 bags

Sugar-free Truvia, 2 tsp.

Grass-fed butter, 1 tbsp.

Full-fat coconut milk, 8 oz.

Chair Blend

Ground nutmeg, 1 tsp.

Pepper, .25 tsp.

Ground cinnamon, 1 tbsp.

Ground cardamom, 2 tsp.

**What you do:**

- Heat the coconut milk and butter in the microwave for two minutes.
- Once hot, add in the tea bags and let it brew for four minutes.
- Discard the tea and add to the blender along with the chai blend and sweetener. Blend for a few seconds until frothy.

## Hash Browns, Bacon, and Eggs

It makes three servings of hash browns, but one serving of eggs and bacon. A single serving of this has 516 calories, 10 g net carbs, 40 g fat, and 27 g protein.

**What you need:**

Hash browns, 2

Slice of bacon

Cooked egg

Hash brown

Melted butter, 1 tbsp.

Pepper

Sea salt, .5 tsp.

Garlic powder, .25 tsp.

Onion powder, .25 tsp.

Egg

Shredded cheese, .75 c

Cauliflower rice, 3 c

**What you do:**

- Add the cauliflower to a bowl and cover with a damp paper towel. Microwave for 2.5 minutes. Allow it to cool slightly.
- Once cooled, place in a cheesecloth and squeeze out as much liquid as you can.
- Place back into the bowl and add in the seasonings, egg, and cheese. Mix everything together.
- Portion the mixture into six rectangles on a baking sheet. Brush them with melted butter.
- Bake for 15 minutes, flip them and then bake for another five. Take them out of the oven and sprinkle with some salt.
- Keep stored in the freezer.
- Heat two up with your bacon and egg for a delicious breakfast.

## Cream Cheese Danish

These can be made in advance and stored in the fridge for a week. Microwave for a few seconds to heat up. This makes four danishes, and each contains 523 calories, 9 g net carbs, 40 g fat, and 19 g protein.

**What you need:**

Baking powder, .5 tsp.

Sea salt, .25 tsp.

Vanilla, .5 tsp.

Egg

Melted butter, 4 tbsp.

Sugar-free Truvia, 2 tbsp.

Almond flour, 6 tbsp.

Coconut flour, 3 tbsp.

Block of mozzarella, 140 grams

Filling

Thawed frozen raspberries or blackberries, .25 c

Sugar-free Truvia, 5 tbsp.

Egg yolk

Vanilla, .5 tsp.

Lemon juice, 1 tsp.

Softened full-fat cream cheese, 6 oz.

**What you do:**

- Mix all of the filling ingredients together, minus the berries. Mix with a hand mixer until light and fluffy. Set in the fridge until ready for use.
- Set your oven to 400. Line a baking sheet with parchment.
- Mix together the coconut flour, almond flour, baking powder, and salt. Mix in the butter, vanilla, and sweetener. Stir until combined.
- Shred the mozzarella. Melt in the microwave for a couple of minutes.
- Mix the cheese into the flour mixture. Once everything is combined, stir in the egg yolk.
- Microwave for 10 seconds and then knead together until combined and is of an even color.
- Roll the dough on the parchment paper and separate into four squares.
- Spoon the filling into the middle of the squares and top with the berries.
- Fold the four corners of the square into the center.
- Bake for 10 to 13 minutes. Pull them out once they are golden in color. They will burn easily.

## Chicken Salad

This makes two servings, and each has 406 calories, 4 g net carbs, 28 g fat, and 31 g protein.

**What you need:**

Salt, .5 tsp.

Butterhead lettuce, 1 head

Garlic powder, .25 tsp.

Onion powder, .25 tsp.

Sour cream, .25 c

Mayonnaise, 2 tbsp.

Thinly sliced celery, 1 stalk

Shredded cheddar cheese, .25 c

Chopped, cooked bacon, 2 slices

Cubed or shredded chicken, 1 c

**What you do:**

- Mix all of the ingredients, except for the lettuce, together. Serve the chicken mixture over the lettuce.

## Lasagna Bowls

This is a single serving recipe and contains 620 calories, 7 g net carbs, 51 g fat, and 30 g protein.

**What you need:**

Italian seasoning, .25 tsp.

Pepper

Salt, .25 tsp.

Parmesan cheese, 2 tbsp.

Mozzarella, 2 tbsp.

Full-fat ricotta cheese, .25 c

Marinara sauce, .25 c

Cooked Italian sausage, 4 oz.

**What you do:**

- Add the sausage to a microwave-safe bowl.

- Drop in the ricotta and sprinkle on the seasonings. Pour in the marinara sauce and top with the remaining cheeses.

- Microwave for two minutes until hot and bubbly.

## Broccoli Cheddar Soup

This makes two servings, and each contains 53 calories, 4 g net carbs, 46 g fat, and 25 g protein.

**What you need:**

Chopped broccoli florets, 1.5 c

Olive oil, 1 tbsp.

Minced garlic, 2 cloves

Sea salt, 1 tsp.

Pepper, .25 tsp.

Chicken brother, 1.75 c

Heavy cream, .5 c

Shredded cheddar cheese, 1.5 c

**What you do:**

- Add the olive oil and garlic to a pot and sauté until fragrant.
- Add in the broccoli florets, broth, and cream. Bring to a boil, reduce heat, and simmer until tender. The time this take will vary on how small the broccoli is, but it should be around 10 to 20 minutes.
- Slowly stir in the shredded cheese. Make sure you stir constantly. Don't add the cheese all at once, slowly add it in so that it melts correctly.

- Once the cheese has melted, remove from heat. This can be stored in the fridge or freezer.

## Chicken Cordon Bleu Casserole

This can be made in advance and stored in the fridge or freezer until needed. It makes four servings, and each contains: 574 calories, 3 g net carbs, 34 g fat, and 59 g protein.

**What you need:**

Minced garlic, 2 cloves

Dijon mustard, 2 tsp.

Sliced Swiss cheese, 3 oz.

Melted butter, .25 c + 1 tbsp.

Softened full-fat cream cheese, 3 oz.

Sliced ham, 3 oz.

Sliced or cubed chicken, 1 lb.

Sea salt, 1 tsp.

Lemon juice, 3 tbsp.

Diced onion, .25 c

**What you do:**

- Set your oven to 350 and grease a 9-inch baking dish.
- Add the onion and butter to a pan. Cook until they are translucent, about five minutes. Stir in the garlic and cook until fragrant.
- In a blender, mix together the salt, lemon juice, Dijon, cream cheese, and butter until smooth.
- Add the chicken to the baking dish, add in the onion mixture, and then the ham. Spread over the sauce.
- Lay the Swiss cheese on top and let it bake for 35 minutes.
- Turn up to the broiler and bake for two minutes until bubbly and golden. Allow it to sit for a few minutes before serving.

# Butter Salmon

This makes two servings, and one serving has 532 calories, 1 g net carbs, 29 g fat, and 65 g protein.

**What you need:**

Salt, 1 tsp.

Pepper, .25 tsp.

Capers, 1 tbsp.

Minced garlic, 2 cloves

Lemon zest, .5 tsp.

Lemon juice, 1 tbsp.

Butter, 3 tbsp.

Salmon fillets, 2

Paprika, .25 tsp.

**What you do:**

- Set your oven to 400.
- Add the butter and garlic to a large skillet. Cook until it becomes fragrant. Add in the lemon zest and juice.
- Add the salmon to the pan and sprinkle with paprika, pepper, and salt.
- Bake until the salmon is cooked all the way through, around 15 minutes. Around five minutes before it is done, add in the capers and add bake to the oven. Serve with the cheesy zucchini gratin.

# Cheesy Zucchini Gratin

This makes two servings, each serving has 298 calories, 6 g net carbs, 25 g fat, and 12 g protein.

**What you need:**

Pepper, .25 tsp.

Sea salt, 1 tsp.

Shredded pepper jack cheese, .75 c

Butter, 1 tbsp.

Heavy cream, .25 c

Minced garlic, 3 cloves

Sliced onion

Zucchini rounds, 2 c

**What you do:**

- Set your oven to 375. Grease an 8-inch baking pan.
- Add a third of the zucchini and the sliced onion in the baking pan and sprinkle with some salt and pepper. Top with a quarter cup of shredded cheese.
- Repeat these layers two more times until you have used all of the onion and zucchini.
- Melt the butter and stir in the garlic until fragrant. Pour this into the heavy cream. Allow to simmer.
- Pour this over the veggies. Place in the oven and bake until it has turned golden and thickened about 35 to 40 minutes.

## Beef Stroganoff Meatballs with Noodles

This makes three servings, and each serving contains 492 calories, 14 g net carbs, 39 g fat, and 19 g protein.

**What you need:**

Garlic powder, .5 tsp.

Pepper, .25 tsp.

Almond flour, 3 tbsp.

Egg

Ground beef, .5 lb.

Sea salt, 1 tsp.

Worcestershire sauce, 1 tsp.

Dried parsley, .5 tsp.

Onion powder, .5 tsp.

Sauce

Konjac noodles, 2 servings

Xanthan gum, pinch

Pepper, .25 tsp.

Sea salt, 1 tsp.

Sour cream, .33 c

Beef broth, .75 c

Minced garlic, 3 cloves

Sliced onion, 1 med

Sliced mushrooms, 8 oz.

Butter, 2 tbsp.

**What you do:**

- Set your oven to 400. Place parchment on a baking sheet.
- Mix all of the meatball ingredients together and use an ice cream scoop to shape it into balls. Place them on the baking sheet. Bake for 10 minutes.
- Meanwhile, add the butter to a pan. Add in the onions and cook until translucent. Add in the mushrooms and cook for seven minutes. Mix in the garlic until fragrant.
- Add the broth, xanthan gum, pepper, salt, and sour cream. Allow this mixture to come to a simmer.
- Add in the cooked meatballs. Place a lid on the pan and allow it to simmer for 20 minutes.
- Serve this over top of konjac noodles.

## Broccoli Cheddar Tots

This makes two servings, and each contains 319 calories, 7 g net carbs, 22 g fat, and 21 g protein.

**What you need:**

Cooking spray

Sea salt, 1 tsp.

Almond flour, .25 c

Coconut flour, 2 tbsp.

Diced onion, .25 c

Parmesan, .25 c

Sharp cheddar cheese, .5 c

Eggs, 2

Broccoli florets, 2 c

**What you do:**

- Set your oven to 400 and line a baking sheet with parchment paper.
- Place the broccoli in a microwave-safe and cover with a damp towel. Microwave two minutes.
- Chop up the broccoli and then add back to the bowl. Add in the rest of the ingredients and combine completely.
- With a tablespoon scoop, portion out the broccoli into tot forms.
- Place the tots on a baking sheet and spray them with cooking spray and bake for six minutes. Flip, and bake for seven minutes.

## Mocha Bonbons

This will make 15 bonbons, and each of the bonbons contains 112 calories, 2.6 g net carbs, 13.4 g fat, and 6 g protein.

**What you need:**

Coffee beans, 15 pieces

Cocoa butter, 2 tbsp.

MCT oil, 3 tbsp.

Dark chocolate chips, .66 c

Cocoa, 2 tbsp.

Sugar-free Truvia, .25 c

Strong coffee, .25 c

Softened full-fat cream cheese, 8 oz.

**What you do:**

- Add the cream cheese to a bowl along with the cocoa, sweetener, and coffee. Blend with an electric mixer until fluffy and combined. Chill for four hours or overnight.

- With a small cookie scoop, scoop the mixture into balls on wax paper. Let them freeze for half an hour.

- Melt the chocolate with the cocoa butter and MCT oil in the microwave. Cover the truffles with the chocolate and top with a single coffee bean. Freeze for an hour, and store in an airtight container.

## Peppermint Mocha Drops

This will make six drops, and each contains 183 calories, 3 g net carbs, 19 g fat, and 0 g protein.

**What you need:**

Vanilla, .5 tsp.

Peppermint extract, 2 tsp.

Liquid stevia, 40 drops

Melted dark chocolate baking chips, .33 c

Softened butter, .25 c

Softened coconut oil, .25 c

**What you do:**

- Place all of the ingredients in a blender and combine until smooth and homogenous.

- Scoop the mixture into small silicon baking cups, should be about two tablespoons of the mixture.

- Freeze until hard, about 15 minutes, and keep stored in the fridge or the freezer.

- When you want, blend into a cup of hot coffee.

## Peanut Butter Cup Smoothie

This makes two servings and per serving contains 486 calories, 6 g net carbs, 30 g protein, and 40 g fat.

**What you need:**

- Peanut butter, 2 tbsp.
- Chocolate protein powder, 1 scoop
- Coconut cream, .75 c
- Water, 1 c
- Ice cubes, 3

**What you do:**

- Place all of the ingredients in a strong blender and mix everything together until smooth.
- Pour the mixture into two glasses.

## Breakfast Bake

This makes eight servings, and each serving contains 303 calories, 3 g net carbs, 24 g fat, and 17 g protein.

**What you need:**

- Shredded cheddar cheese, .5 c
- Pepper
- Salt

- Chopped oregano, 1 tbsp.
- Cooked spaghetti squash, 2 c
- Eggs, 8
- Sausage, 1 lb.
- Olive oil, 1 tbsp.

**What you do:**

- Set your oven to 375 and grease a 9 x 13 casserole dish.
- Add the olive oil to a large ovenproof skillet and heat up.
- Add the sausage and cook thoroughly around five minutes. As the sausage is cooking, beat the eggs together along with the oregano and squash. Season it with some pepper and salt.
- Mix the sausage into the egg mixture. Stir everything together until combined and pour into your prepared casserole dish.
- Sprinkle the top with the cheese and cover it loosely with foil.
- Slide the casserole into the oven for 30 minutes, and then take the foil off and let it cook for another 15 minutes.
- Allow to stand for ten minutes before you serve it.

# Mushroom Frittata

This makes six servings, and each serving contains 316 calories, 1 g net carbs, 27 g fat, and 16 g protein.

**What you need:**

- Pepper
- Salt
- Crumbled goat cheese, .5 c
- Beaten eggs, 10
- Chopped and cooked bacon, 6 slices
- Shredded spinach, 1 c
- Sliced mushrooms, 1 c
- Olive oil, 2 tbsp.

**What you do:**

- Start by placing your oven to 350.
- Heat the olive oil in a large ovenproof pan.
- Sauté the mushrooms until they are browned lightly, around three minutes.
- Add the bacon and spinach to the pan and sauté until the greens have wilted.
- Add the beaten eggs. Don't stir. Allow the eggs to set, and life the edges up every so often to let the uncooked egg to flow underneath. Cook for around three to four minutes.

- Sprinkle goat cheese on top and season with some pepper and salt.
- Bake the frittata until it has fully set and browned, about 15 minutes.
- Remove and allow to sit for five minutes. Slice into six wedges and serve.

## Avocado and Eggs

This makes four servings, and each serving contains 324 calories, 3 g net carbs, 25 g fat, 19 g protein.

**What you need:**
- Pepper
- Salt
- Cheddar cheese, .25 c
- Cooked and shredded chicken breast, 4 oz.
- Eggs, 4
- Avocados, 2

**What you do:**
- Start by placing the oven to 425.
- Slice the avocados in half and remove the pits. Scoop out a bit of the flesh from the avocado so that it is about twice as big as it was.
- Lay the halves into an 8-inch square baking dish with the fleshy side up.
- Crack on egg into each of the holes in the avocado halves. Divide the shredded chicken between the halves and sprinkle the tops of them with cheese. Season them with a little bit of pepper and salt.
- Slide them into the oven and cook until the eggs are cooked to your desired doneness, about 15 to 20 minutes.

## Creamy Cinnamon Smoothie

This makes two servings, and each serving contains 492 calories, 6 g net carbs, 47 g fat, and 18 g protein.

**What you need:**

- Vanilla, .5 tsp.
- Ground cinnamon, 1 tsp.
- Liquid stevia, 5 drops
- Vanilla protein powder, 1 scoop
- Coconut milk, 2 c

**What you do:**

- Add all of the ingredients to your blender and mix until everything is smooth and incorporated.
- Divide the mixture between two glasses.

## Everything Bagel

This makes 12 servings, and each serving contains 25 calories, .5 g net carbs, 2 g fat, 3 g protein.

**What you need:**

- Everything bagel seasoning
- Smoked salmon, 4 oz.
- Full-fat butter, 1 tbsp.
- Full-fat cream cheese, 4 oz.

**What you do:**

- Mix together the salmon, butter, and cream cheese together until it is evenly distributed. You don't want to have clumps of each ingredient. You want everything to be smooth.

- Place in the refrigerator for 30 minutes. Allow the mixture to stiffen up a bit.

- Once it has become firmer, divide the mixture into 12 equal portions and roll into balls.

- Finally, roll the balls in some of the everything bagel seasonings. If you don't want to use salmon, you can also use bacon.

- When you keep them refrigerated, the bagels will keep a firmer consistency and are easy to grab in the morning when you don't have time to cook.

## Nut Medley Granola

This makes eight serving, and each serving contains 391 calories, 4 g net carbs, 38 g fat, and 10 g protein.

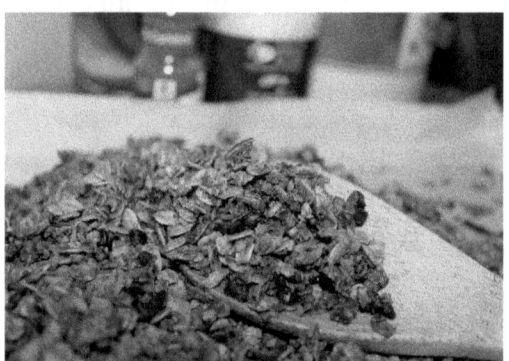

**What you need:**

- Ground nutmeg, .5 tsp.

- Ground cinnamon, 1 tsp.

- Liquid Stevia, 10 drops

- Melted coconut oil, .5 c, melted

- Walnuts, .5 c

- Pumpkin seeds, .5 c, raw
- Sunflower seeds, 1 c, raw
- Shredded unsweetened coconut, 2 c
- Sliced almonds, 1 c

**What you do:**

- Heat up your oven to 250 degrees. Take two large baking sheets and line them with parchment paper. Set this to the side.
- Add the walnuts, pumpkin seeds, sunflower seeds, almonds, and shredded coconut to a large bowl and toss until mixed well.
- Add the nutmeg, cinnamon, stevia, and coconut oil to a small bowl and mix until well blended.
- Pour this mixture over the nuts and seeds. Using your hands toss the nuts until they have been well coated with the coconut mixture.
- Divide the granola between the two baking sheets and spread evenly.
- Bake for one hour. Stir the granola every 15 minutes until crunchy and golden.
- Remove from oven and allow to cool. Break up any large chunks into bite-size pieces.
- Store in an airtight container. This can be stored in the freezer or refrigerator for one month.

## Berry Green Smoothie

This makes two servings, and each serving contains 436 calories, 6 g net carbs, 36 g fat, and 28 g protein.

**What you need:**

- Vanilla protein powder, 1 scoop
- Coconut oil, 1 tbsp.
- Cream cheese, .75 c
- Kale, .5 c, shredded
- Raspberries, .5 tsp.
- Water, 1 c

**What you do:**

- Place all ingredients into the blender. Blend until smooth and creamy.
- Pour into glasses and enjoy.

# Bacon Artichoke Omelet

This makes four servings, and each serving contains 435 calories, 3 g net carbs, 39 g fat, and 17 g protein.

**What you need:**

- Pepper
- Salt
- Artichoke hearts, .5 c, canned, packed in water
- Onion, .25 c, chopped
- Olive oil, 1 tbsp.
- Chopped bacon, 8 slices
- Heavy whipping cream, 2 tbsp.
- Eggs, 6 beaten

**What you do:**

- Heat up a large skillet and cook the bacon until it is crispy.
- Remove bacon and drain. Allow to cool for a few minutes.
- Put heavy cream, bacon, and eggs into a bowl and whisk until well blended. Set to the side.
- Remove bacon grease from pan and wipe clean. Add olive oil and onion and cook until tender. This will take about three minutes.
- Pour the egg mixture into the skillet and swirl it around for one minute.
- Continue to cook, lifting the edges to allow the uncooked egg to glow under for about two minutes.
- Put the artichoke hearts on top and flip the omelet. Cook an additional four minutes until the egg is firm. Flip again so that the artichoke hearts are back on top.

- Take off heat, cut into quarters and season generously with pepper and salt. Place on plates and enjoy.

# Chapter 10: Breakfast

## Peanut Butter Cup Smoothie

This makes two servings and per serving contains 486 calories, 6 g net carbs, 30 g protein, and 40 g fat.

### What you need:

- Peanut butter, 2 tbsp.
- Chocolate protein powder, 1 scoop
- Coconut cream, .75 c
- Water, 1 c
- Ice cubes, 3

### What you do:

- Place all of the ingredients in a strong blender and mix everything together until smooth.
- Pour the mixture into two glasses.

## Breakfast Bake

This makes eight servings, and each serving contains 303 calories, 3 g net carbs, 24 g fat, and 17 g protein.

### What you need:

- Shredded cheddar cheese, .5 c
- Pepper
- Salt

- Chopped oregano, 1 tbsp.
- Cooked spaghetti squash, 2 c
- Eggs, 8
- Sausage, 1 lb.
- Olive oil, 1 tbsp.

## What you do:

- Set your oven to 375 and grease a 9 x 13 casserole dish.
- Add the olive oil to a large ovenproof skillet and heat up.
- Add the sausage and cook thoroughly around five minutes. As the sausage is cooking, beat the eggs together along with the oregano and squash. Season it with some pepper and salt.
- Mix the sausage into the egg mixture. Stir everything together until combined and pour into your prepared casserole dish.
- Sprinkle the top with the cheese and cover it loosely with foil.
- Slide the casserole into the oven for 30 minutes, and then take the foil off and let it cook for another 15 minutes.
- Allow to stand for ten minutes before you serve it.

# Mushroom Frittata

This makes six servings, and each serving contains 316 calories, 1 g net carbs, 27 g fat, and 16 g protein.

## What you need:

- Pepper
- Salt
- Crumbled goat cheese, .5 c
- Beaten eggs, 10
- Chopped and cooked bacon, 6 slices
- Shredded spinach, 1 c
- Sliced mushrooms, 1 c
- Olive oil, 2 tbsp.

## What you do:

- Start by placing your oven to 350.
- Heat the olive oil in a large ovenproof pan.
- Sauté the mushrooms until they are browned lightly, around three minutes.
- Add the bacon and spinach to the pan and sauté until the greens have wilted.

- Add the beaten eggs. Don't stir. Allow the eggs to set, and life the edges up every so often to let the uncooked egg to flow underneath. Cook for around three to four minutes.

- Sprinkle goat cheese on top and season with some pepper and salt.

- Bake the frittata until it has fully set and browned, about 15 minutes.

- Remove and allow to sit for five minutes. Slice into six wedges and serve.

## Avocado and Eggs

This makes four servings, and each serving contains 324 calories, 3 g net carbs, 25 g fat, 19 g protein.

## What you need:

- Pepper
- Salt
- Cheddar cheese, .25 c
- Cooked and shredded chicken breast, 4 oz.
- Eggs, 4
- Avocados, 2

## What you do:

- Start by placing the oven to 425.
- Slice the avocados in half and remove the pits. Scoop out a bit of the flesh from the avocado so that it is about twice as big as it was.
- Lay the halves into an 8-inch square baking dish with the fleshy side up.
- Crack on egg into each of the holes in the avocado halves. Divide the shredded chicken between the halves and sprinkle the tops of them with cheese. Season them with a little bit of pepper and salt.
- Slide them into the oven and cook until the eggs are cooked to your desired doneness, about 15 to 20 minutes.

## Creamy Cinnamon Smoothie

This makes two servings, and each serving contains 492 calories, 6 g net carbs, 47 g fat, and 18 g protein.

### What you need:
- Vanilla, .5 tsp.
- Ground cinnamon, 1 tsp.
- Liquid stevia, 5 drops
- Vanilla protein powder, 1 scoop
- Coconut milk, 2 c

### What you do:
- Add all of the ingredients to your blender and mix until everything is smooth and incorporated.
- Divide the mixture between two glasses.

## Everything Bagel

This makes 12 servings, and each serving contains 25 calories, .5 g net carbs, 2 g fat, 3 g protein.

### What you need:
- Everything bagel seasoning
- Smoked salmon, 4 oz.
- Full-fat butter, 1 tbsp.
- Full-fat cream cheese, 4 oz.

## What you do:

- Mix together the salmon, butter, and cream cheese together until it is evenly distributed. You don't want to have clumps of each ingredient. You want everything to be smooth.

- Place in the refrigerator for 30 minutes. Allow the mixture to stiffen up a bit.

- Once it has become firmer, divide the mixture into 12 equal portions and roll into balls.

- Finally, roll the balls in some of the everything bagel seasonings. If you don't want to use salmon, you can also use bacon.

- When you keep them refrigerated, the bagels will keep a firmer consistency and are easy to grab in the morning when you don't have time to cook.

## Nut Medley Granola

This makes eight serving, and each serving contains 391 calories, 4 g net carbs, 38 g fat, and 10 g protein.

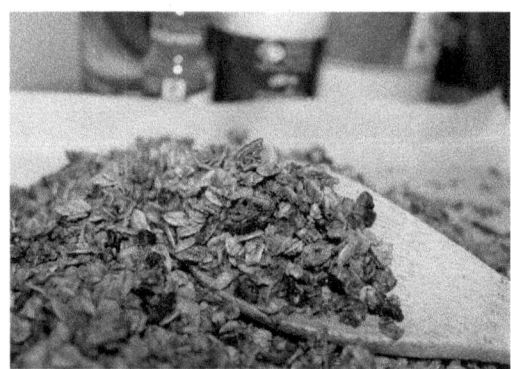

## What you need:

- Ground nutmeg, .5 tsp.

- Ground cinnamon, 1 tsp.

- Liquid Stevia, 10 drops

- Melted coconut oil, .5 c, melted

- Walnuts, .5 c
- Pumpkin seeds, .5 c, raw
- Sunflower seeds, 1 c, raw
- Shredded unsweetened coconut, 2 c
- Sliced almonds, 1 c

## What you do:

- Heat up your oven to 250 degrees. Take two large baking sheets and line them with parchment paper. Set this to the side.
- Add the walnuts, pumpkin seeds, sunflower seeds, almonds, and shredded coconut to a large bowl and toss until mixed well.
- Add the nutmeg, cinnamon, stevia, and coconut oil to a small bowl and mix until well blended.
- Pour this mixture over the nuts and seeds. Using your hands toss the nuts until they have been well coated with the coconut mixture.
- Divide the granola between the two baking sheets and spread evenly.
- Bake for one hour. Stir the granola every 15 minutes until crunchy and golden.
- Remove from oven and allow to cool. Break up any large chunks into bite-size pieces.
- Store in an airtight container. This can be stored in the freezer or refrigerator for one month.

## Berry Green Smoothie

This makes two servings, and each serving contains 436 calories, 6 g net carbs, 36 g fat, and 28 g protein.

### What you need:

- Vanilla protein powder, 1 scoop
- Coconut oil, 1 tbsp.
- Cream cheese, .75 c
- Kale, .5 c, shredded
- Raspberries, .5 tsp.
- Water, 1 c

### What you do:

- Place all ingredients into the blender. Blend until smooth and creamy.
- Pour into glasses and enjoy.

# Bacon Artichoke Omelet

This makes four servings, and each serving contains 435 calories, 3 g net carbs, 39 g fat, and 17 g protein.

## What you need:

- Pepper
- Salt
- Artichoke hearts, .5 c, canned, packed in water
- Onion, .25 c, chopped
- Olive oil, 1 tbsp.
- Chopped bacon, 8 slices
- Heavy whipping cream, 2 tbsp.
- Eggs, 6 beaten

## What you do:

- Heat up a large skillet and cook the bacon until it is crispy.
- Remove bacon and drain. Allow to cool for a few minutes.
- Put heavy cream, bacon, and eggs into a bowl and whisk until well blended. Set to the side.
- Remove bacon grease from pan and wipe clean. Add olive oil and onion and cook until tender. This will take about three minutes.
- Pour the egg mixture into the skillet and swirl it around for one minute.
- Continue to cook, lifting the edges to allow the uncooked egg to glow under for about two minutes.
- Put the artichoke hearts on top and flip the omelet. Cook an additional four minutes until the egg is firm. Flip again so that the artichoke hearts are back on top.

- Take off heat, cut into quarters and season generously with pepper and salt. Place on plates and enjoy.

# Chapter 11: Main Dishes

## Stuffed Chicken Breasts

This makes four servings, and each serving contains 389 calories, 3 g net carbs, 30 g fat, and 25 g protein.

### What you need:

- EVOO, 2 tbsp.
- Skin-on chicken breasts, 4-5 oz. breasts
- Chopped basil, 2 tbsp.
- Chopped roasted red pepper, .25 c
- Chopped kalamata olives, .25 c
- Room temp goat cheese, .5 c
- Chopped sweet onion, .25 c
- Butter, 1 tbsp.

### What you do:

- Start by placing your oven to 400.
- In a small pan, melt the butter and add in the onion. Let the onion cook until tender, around three minutes.
- Place the onion in a bowl and add in the basil, red pepper, olives, and cheese. Stir everything together until it is all well blended. Refrigerate the mixture for at least 30 minutes.
- Slice a horizontal pocket into each of the chicken breasts and stuff each evenly with the filling that you made earlier. Secure them with toothpicks.
- Heat the olive oil in an ovenproof skillet and add in the chicken. Brown the chicken on both sides, about five minutes on each side.
- Slide the skillet into the oven and cook until the chicken has cooked through around 15 minutes. Take out the toothpicks before serving.

# Roasted Pork Loin with Mustard Sauce

This makes eight servings, and each serving contains 368 calories, 2 g net carbs, 29 g fat, and 25 g protein.

## What you need:

- Grainy mustard, 3 tbsp.
- Heavy cream, 1.5 c
- Olive oil, 3 tbsp.
- Pepper
- Salt
- Boneless pork loin roast, 2 lbs.

## What you do:

- Start by placing your oven to 375.
- Rub your pork roast with pepper and salt.
- Add the olive oil to a large skillet. Add in the roast and brown on all sides. This should take about six minutes in total. Place the roast into a baking dish.
- Bake for about an hour, or until the internal temperature reaches 155.
- When there are around 15 minutes left on the roasting time, add a small pot on medium heat and add the mustard and cream.
- Stir the sauce until it comes to a simmer. Turn the heat to low and allow it to simmer for five minutes, or until it becomes thick. Take the pot off the heat.
- Allow the pork to rest for ten minutes. Slice and serve topped with the sauce.

## Garlic-Braised Short Rib

This makes four servings, and each serving contains 481 calories, 2 g net carbs, 38 g fat, and 29 g protein.

## What you need:

- Beef stock, 3 c
- Dry red wine, .5 c
- Minced garlic, 2 tsp.
- Olive oil, 1 tbsp.
- Pepper
- Salt
- Beef short ribs, 4-4 oz. racks

## What you do:

- Start by placing your oven to 325. Rub the ribs with pepper and salt.
- Grab a deep ovenproof skillet and add in the olive oil and let heat to medium-high.
- Sear the ribs in the pan on all sides until they are browned. Transfer to a plate.

- Place the garlic in a skillet and cook until fragrant, around three minutes.

- Whisk the wine to deglaze your pan. Make sure that you scrap all of the little-browned bits off of the bottom of the pan. Let the wine simmer until it has reduced slightly, about two minutes.

- Pour in the beef stock, and then add the ribs and any juices they have accumulated. Allow the mixture to come to a boil.

- Place a lid on the skillet and place it in the oven. Cook the ribs for about two hours. They should be fall-off-the-bone tender.

- Serve the ribs along with the cooking liquid drizzled over.

## Italian Beef Burgers

This makes four servings, and each serving contains 441 calories, 3 g net carbs, 37 g fat, and 22 g protein.

### What you need:

- Thinly sliced onion, .25 onion
- Tomato sliced into four slices
- Olive oil, 1 tbsp.
- Salt, .25 tsp.
- Minced garlic, 1 tsp.
- Chopped basil, 2 tbsp.
- Ground almonds, .25 c
- Lean ground beef, 1 lb.

### What you do:

- Combine the salt, garlic, basil, ground almonds, and ground beef together in a bowl.

- Form the mixture into four equal sized patties and flatten them to about a half-inch thick.

- Add olive oil to a large skillet and heat to medium-high.

- Panfry the burger patties until they are cooked through; flip them once during the cooking time. It should take about six minutes on each side.

- Pay away excess grease and serve along with onion and tomato.

## Sirloin with Compound Butter

This makes four servings, and each serving contains 544 calories, 0 g net carbs, 44 g fat, and 35 g protein.

## What you need:

- Pepper

- Salt

- Olive oil, 1 tbsp.

- Beef sirloin steaks, 4-5 oz.

- Blue cheese, 4 oz.

- Room temp butter, 6 tbsp.

## What you do:

- Add the butter to a blender and pulse until it has been whipped up, around two minutes.

- Add in the cheese, and pulse until well mixed.

- Spoon out on a sheet of plastic wrap and roll it into a log that is about 1.5 inches in diameter.

- Refrigerate until it has set up, around an hour.

- Slice into half inch disks and place on a plate in the refrigerator until you are ready to serve your steaks. Store any of the leftovers in the fridge for up to a week.

- Heat up your grill. As this is happening, allow the steaks to come up to room temp.

- Rub the steaks with olive oil, pepper, and salt.

- Grill the steaks until they are done to your likely. Six minutes on each side will cook it to around medium. If you don't have a grill, you can pan fry or broil the steaks for about seven minutes on each side for medium.

- Allow the steaks to rest for about ten minutes. Serve each steak along with a disk of the butter.

## Lamb with Tomato Pesto

This makes eight servings, and each serving contains 352 calories, 3 g net carbs, 29 g fat, and 17 g protein.

### What you need:

- Lamb
- Olive oil, 2 tbsp.
- Pepper
- Salt
- Leg of lamb, 2 lb.
- Pesto
- Minced garlic, 2 tsp.
- Chopped basil, 2 tbsp.
- EVOO, 2 tbsp.
- Pine nuts, .25 c
- Sun-dried tomatoes in oil, drained, 1 c

## What you do:

- For the Pesto – Add the garlic, basil, olive oil, pine nuts, and tomatoes to a blender or food processor. Mix up until smooth and then set aside until you need to use it.

- Leg of Lamb – Start by placing your oven to 400. Rub the lamb with pepper and salt.

- Add olive oil to an ovenproof pan and heat to medium-high.

- Sear the lamb on all sides until it is nicely browned.

- Spread the tomato peas over the lamb and set on a baking sheet. Slide into the oven and roast until it reaches your desired doneness. An hour of cooking will take it to about medium.

- Allow the lamb to rest for ten minutes before you serve it.

## Lamb Chops with Kalamata Tapenade

This makes four servings, and each serving contains 348 calories, 1 g net carbs, 28 g fat, and 21 g protein.

## What you need:

- Lamb Chops
- Olive oil, 1 tbsp.
- Pepper
- Salt
- French-cut lamb chops, 2 1-lb. racks
- Tapenade
- Lemon juice, 2 tsp.
- Minced garlic, 2 tsp.
- EVOO, 2 tbsp.

- Chopped parsley, 2 tbsp.
- Kalamata olives, 1 c

## What you do:

- For the Tapenade – Add the lemon juice, garlic, olive oil, parsley, and olives to a food processor and process until is pureed, but still chunky.
- Transfer to a container and keep in the fridge until you need it.
- For the Lamb Chops – Start by placing your oven on 450. Rub the lamb with pepper and salt.
- Place the oil in an ovenproof skillet and heat up to medium-high. Place the lamb racks on the pan and sear until browned on all sides.
- Place the racks upright in the skillet. The bones should be interlaced. Roast them in the oven until it has reached your desired doneness. For medium-rare, cook it for about 20 minutes. The internal temp needs to reach at least 125.
- Allow the lamb to rest for at least ten minutes. Slice the lamb racks into individual chops. Give four chops per person and top with the tapenade you made earlier.

# Herb Butter Scallops

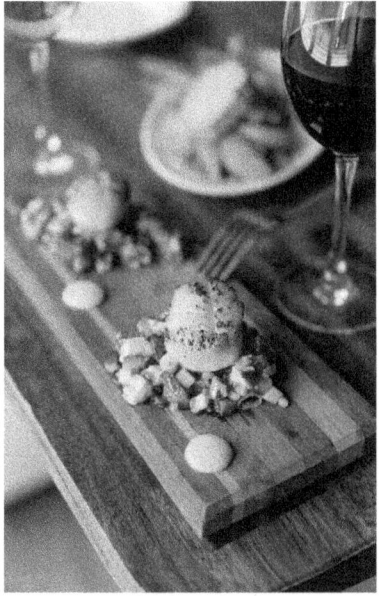

This makes four servings, and each serving contains 306 calories, 4 g net carbs, 24 g fat, and 19 g protein.

## What you need:

- Chopped basil, 2 tsp.
- Butter, 8 tbsp.
- Pepper
- Chopped thyme, 1 tsp.
- Minced garlic, 2 tsp.
- One lemon juiced
- Cleaned sea scallops, 1 lb.

## What you do:

- Make sure the scallops are completely dry by patting them with paper towels. Season with pepper.
- Warm a large skillet and add two tablespoons butter to skillet.

- Evenly space the scallops in the skillet. Cook on each side until golden brown. This will take about 2 ½ minutes for each side.

- Remove from skillet onto a plate and set to the side.

- Add the rest of the butter to the skillet and add garlic, sauté for three minutes until garlic is fragrant and translucent.

- Add in thyme, basil, and lemon juice, stir well. Put the scallops back into the skillet. Flip them over to coat with sauce.

- Serve and enjoy.

## Halibut with Citrus Butter Sauce

This makes four servings, and each serving contains 319 calories, 2 g net carbs, 26 g fat, and 22 g protein.

### What you need:

- Olive oil, 2 tbsp.
- Chopped parsley, 2 tsp.
- Orange juice, 1 tbsp.
- Lemon juice, 1 tbsp.
- Dry white wine, 3 tbsp.
- Minced shallot, 1
- Minced garlic, 2 tsp.
- Butter, .25 c
- Pepper
- Halibut fillets, 4-5 oz. fillets

### What you do:

- Make sure the fish is completely dry by patting it with paper towels. Season the fillet with pepper and salt. Place on a plate that has been lined with paper towels.

- Warm a saucepan and melt the butter.
- Add in shallot and garlic and cook until tender. This will take three minutes.
- Add in the orange juice, lemon juice, and white wine and allow the sauce to simmer. Let it cook until it is slightly thickened. This will take about two minutes.
- Take off heat and add in parsley. Set to the side.
- Warm a large skillet and add olive oil.
- Fry the fish until lightly browned and cooked through, turning over once. This will take about ten minutes.
- Place each piece of fish on a plate. Put a spoonful of sauce on each fillet.

## Coconut Haddock

This makes four servings, and each serving contains 299 calories, 1 g net carbs, 24 g fat, and 20 g protein.

### What you need:

- Melted coconut oil, 2 tbsp.
- Ground hazelnuts, .25 c
- Unsweetened shredded coconut, 1 c
- Pepper
- Salt
- Boneless haddock fillets, 4-5 oz.

### What you do:

- Heat up your oven to 400. Put parchment paper onto a large baking sheet. Set to the side.
- Make sure the fillets are dry by patting them with paper towels. Season them with pepper and salt.
- Put the hazelnuts and coconut into a small bowl and stir to mix well.

- Place the fish fillets into the coconut mixture. Make sure both sides of the fish are coated well.
- Put the fish on the prepared baking sheet and brush both sides with coconut oil.
- Bake for 12 minutes or until the topping is golden brown and flakes easily.
- Serve and enjoy.

# Chapter 12: Side Dishes

## Asparagus and Walnuts

This makes four servings, and each serving contains 124 calories, 2 g net carbs, 12 g fat, and 3 g protein.

### What you need:

- Chopped walnuts, .25 c
- Pepper
- Salt
- Trimmed asparagus, .75 lb.
- Olive oil, 1.5 tbsp.

### What you do:

- Heat a large skillet with some olive oil over medium-high.
- Add the asparagus and sauté until they are tender and browned lightly. This takes about five minutes.
- Season with some pepper and salt.
- Take the pan off the heat and toss the walnuts in with the asparagus.

# Creamed Spinach

This makes four servings, and each serving contains 195 calories, 1 g net carbs, 20 g fat, and 3 g protein.

## What you need:

- Nutmeg, pinch
- Pepper
- Salt
- Herbed chicken stock, .25 c
- Heavy cream, .75 c
- Stemmed and cleaned spinach, 4 c
- Sliced onion, .5
- Butter, 1 tbsp.

## What you do:

- Add the butter to a large pan. Add in the onion and sauté until lightly browned around five minutes.
- Mix in the nutmeg, pepper, salt, chicken stock, heavy cream, and spinach.
- Cook for about five minutes, or until the spinach has wilted.
- Continue to cook until the spinach is tender and the sauce has thickened, 15 minutes.

# Golden Rosti

This makes eight servings, and each serving contains 171 calories, 3 g net carbs, 15 g fat, and 5 g protein.

## What you need:

- Butter, 2 tbsp.
- Pepper
- Salt
- Chopped thyme, 1 tsp.
- Minced garlic, 2 tsp.
- Grated parmesan, 2 tbsp.
- Shredded raw celeriac, 1 c
- Shredded acorn squash, 1 c
- Chopped bacon, 8 slices

## What you do:

- Heat up a large skillet and cook the bacon until it is crispy.
- As the bacon cooks, combines the thyme, garlic, parmesan, celeriac, and squash. Season it with a generous amount of pepper and salt. Set to the side.
- Take the bacon out of the pan with a slotted spoon and add to the rosti mixture. Stir everything together.
- Keep two tablespoons of bacon fat in the skillet and add in the butter.
- Turn the heat down and add the rosti mixture to the skillet and spread it out so that it forms a large round patty that is about an inch thick.
- Cook until the bottom has turned golden and has crisped up.
- Flip it over and let it cook until the other side is crispy and it is cooked in the middle.
- Take it out of the pan and slice into eight pieces.

## Mushrooms with Camembert

This makes four servings, and each serving contains 161 calories, 3 g net carbs, 13 g fat, and 9 g protein.

### What you need:

- Pepper
- Diced camembert cheese, 4 oz.
- Halved button mushrooms, 1 lb.
- Minced garlic, 2 tsp.
- Butter, 2 tbsp.

### What you do:

- Melt the butter in a large skillet on medium-high.
- Cook the garlic until it becomes fragrant, about three minutes. Add in the mushrooms and cook until tender, about ten minutes. Mix in the cheese. Sauté for two minutes, or until the cheese has melted.
- Stir in some pepper and enjoy.

## Crispy Zucchini

This makes four servings, and each serving contains 94 calories, 1 g net carbs, 8 g fat, and 4 g protein.

### What you need:

- Pepper
- Grated parmesan, .5 c

- Zucchini sliced into .25-inch rounds, 4 zucchini
- Butter, 2 tbsp.

## What you do:

- Melt the butter in a large skillet.
- Add in the zucchini and let it cook until it is tender and browned, around five minutes.
- Spread the zucchini evenly onto the bottom of the skillet and sprinkle the top of the veggies with the parmesan. Enjoy.

## Cheesy Cauliflower

This makes four servings, and each serving contains 183 calories, 4 g net carbs, 15 g fat, and 8 g protein.

## What you need:

- Pepper
- Salt
- Room temp butter, 2 tbsp.
- Heavy cream, .25 c
- Shredded cheddar, .5 c
- Roughly chopped cauliflower, 1 head

## What you do:

- Add water to a pot and fill three-quarters full. Place on high and bring to boil.
- Add the cauliflower and blanch until tender, around five minutes. Drain the cauliflower.
- Place the cauliflower in a food processor and add in the butter, cream, and cheese. Puree the mixture until it is whipped and creamy.
- Season to taste with pepper and salt.

## Cheesy Bacon Deviled Eggs

This makes 12 servings, and each serving contains 85 calories, 2 g net carbs, 7 g fat, and 6 g protein.

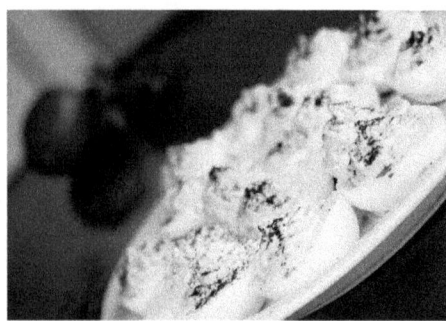

## What you need:

- Chopped and cooked bacon, 6 slices
- Pepper
- Salt
- Dijon mustard, .5 tsp.
- Shredded Swiss cheese, .25 tsp.
- Chopped avocado, .25
- Mayonnaise, .25 c
- Hardboiled eggs, 6

## What you do:

- Cut the eggs in half lengthwise.
- Remove the yolks carefully and put them in a bowl. Set the whites onto a plate.
- Using a fork and mash the yolks. Add in the mustard, cheese, avocado, and mayonnaise. Stir well until blended. Season with pepper and salt.
- Carefully spoon the yolk mixture into each egg white. Add chopped bacon onto the top of each egg.

- If not eating immediately, store them in an airtight container in the refrigerator for no longer than one day.

# Chapter 13: Desserts, Fat Bombs, and Extras

## Doughnut Holes

This makes eight servings, and each serving contains 142 calories, 6.2 g net carbs, 14.1 g fat, and 0 g protein.

### What you need:

- Vanilla extract, 1 tsp.
- Coconut flour, 1 tbsp.
- Coconut oil, 2 tbsp.
- Stevie, 2 tbsp.
- Hot water, 2 oz.
- Softened coconut butter, 4 oz.

### What you do:

- Set aside one tablespoon of sweetener. Place all of the rest of the ingredients into a mixer and combine until mixed thoroughly.
- Place into the freezer for 30 minutes to allow it to set up.
- Once it has hardened, divide it into eight portions and roll them into balls.

- Add the reserved sweetener into a food processor and blend until it turns into powder.
- Roll the balls into the powder and enjoy.

## Chocolate-Coconut Treats

This makes 16 servings, and each serving contains 43 calories, 1 g net carbs, 5 g fat, and 1 g protein.

### What you need:
- Shredded unsweetened coconut, .25 c
- Salt
- Liquid stevia, 4 drops
- Unsweetened cocoa powder, .25 c
- Coconut oil, .33 c

### What you do:
- Place some parchment paper in a 6-inch square baking dish and set aside.
- In a pot, add in the salt, stevia, cocoa, and coconut oil. Stir everything together for about three minutes.
- Mix in the coconut and press the mixture into the prepared baking dish.
- Place in the fridge until it has hardened, around 30 minutes.
- Cut into 16 equal squares and keep stored in a cool place.

## Herbed Avocado Butter

This makes two cups, and one tablespoon contains 22 calories, 1 g net carbs, 2 g fat, and 0 g protein.

### What you need:

- Pepper
- Salt
- Minced garlic, 1 tsp.
- Chopped basil, 1 tsp.
- Chopped cilantro, 2 tsp.
- Lemon juice, .5 of a lemon
- Quartered avocado, 1
- Room temp butter, .25 c

### What you do:

- Add the garlic, basil, cilantro, lemon juice, avocado, and butter to a food processor and mix up until it is smooth.
- Season with some pepper and salt.
- Place the butter on a sheet of wax paper and roll the compound butter into a log share. Place this back in the fridge until it is firm, around four hours.
- You can use this on chicken, fish, or steak. Keep stored, wrapped tightly, in the freezer for a week.

## Mayonnaise

This makes four cups, and two tablespoons contain 61 calories, 0 g net carbs, 7 g fat, and 0 g protein.

### What you need:

- Pepper
- Salt

- Lemon juice, .25 c
- EVOO, 1.5 c
- Dijon mustard, 2 tbsp.
- Eggs, 2

## What you do:

- By Hand – place the mustard and eggs in a large bowl and whisk together until they are well combined, around two minutes.
- Pour the oil into the eggs in a continuous thin stream as you continue to whisk. Do this until the mayonnaise is thick and emulsified.
- Add in the lemon juice and whisk together and blended. Season with some pepper and salt.
- With a Food Processor – add the mustard and eggs in a food processor and blend until smooth.
- With the processor running, slowly drizzle in the oil, mixing until the mayonnaise is thick and emulsified.
- Add in the lemon juice until smooth and season with some salt and pepper.

## Peanut Butter Cups

This makes six servings, and each serving contains: 231 calories, 3 g net carbs, 15.1 g fat, and 2 g protein.

## What you need:

- Vanilla, .25 tsp.
- Stevia, .5 tsp.
- Cocoa powder, 1 tbsp.
- Unsweetened baker's chocolate, 1 oz.
- Coconut oil, .25 c

- Peanut butter, .25 c

### What you do:

- In a pot, add the baker's chocolate and allow it to melt.

- Mix in the peanut butter. The softer it is, the easier it will be to mix in. Stir in the cocoa powder and coconut oil until it is thoroughly mixed.

- Using paper or silicone cupcake liners, pour the mixture into six cupcake molds.

- Allow them to freeze for an hour to let it solidify. Once hard, you can take them out of the liners and store them, or leave them in the liners until you want to eat them. Keep them stored in the fridge.

## Peanut Butter Mousse

This makes four servings, and each serving contains 280 calories, 3 g net carbs, 28 g fat, and 6 g protein.

### What you need:

- Liquid stevia, 4 drops

- Vanilla, 1 tsp.

- Peanut butter, .25 c

- Heavy cream, 1 c

### What you do:

- Using a medium bowl, beat the peanut butter, heavy cream, stevia, and vanilla together until they form stiff peaks. This takes about five minutes.

- Spoon the mousse into four bowls and refrigerate for at last 30 minutes before you serve.

## Strawberry Butter

This makes three cups, and each tablespoon contains 23 calories, 1 g net carbs, 2 g fat, and 0 g protein.

### What you need:

- Vanilla, 1 tsp.
- Fresh lemon juice, .5 tbsp.
- Fresh strawberries, .75 c
- Coconut oil, 1 tbsp.
- Shredded unsweetened coconut, 2 c

### What you do:

- Place the coconut in a food processor and puree it until it becomes smooth and buttery. This will take about 15 minutes.
- Add in the vanilla, lemon juice, strawberries, and coconut oil to the coconut mixture. Process this until smooth. You will want to scrape the sides of the bowl down.
- Pour the butter through a fine sieve to get rid of the strawberry seeds. You can use the back of a spoon to help push the butter through.
- Place the strawberry butter in an airtight container and keep it refrigerated. It will last for at least two weeks.
- This is great served on fish or chicken.

## Balsamic Dressing

This makes one cup, and each tablespoon contains 83 calories, 0 g net carbs, 9 g fat, and 0 g protein.

### What you need:

- Pepper
- Salt
- Minced garlic, 1 tsp.
- Chopped basil, 1 tsp.
- Chopped oregano, 2 tbsp.
- Balsamic vinegar, .25 c
- EVOO, 1 c

### What you do:

- Add the vinegar and olive oil to a bowl and whisk it together until they are well emulsified. This takes about three minutes.
- Whisk in the garlic, basil, and oregano until it is well combined, around one minute.
- Add in the pepper and salt to your taste.
- Pour into an airtight container. This can be stored in the refrigerator for up to a week. Before you use it, shake it well.

# Hollandaise

This makes two cups, and each tablespoon contains 173 calories, 1 g net carbs, 17 g fat, and 5 g protein.

## What you need:

- Salt
- Lemon juice, 4 tsp.
- Cold water, 2 tsp.
- Egg yolks, 4
- Unsalted butter, 1.5 c

## What you do:

- Melt the butter in a heavy-bottomed pot on low heat.
- Take the pot off the heat and allow the butter to cool for five minutes.
- Carefully skim the foam from the top of the cooled butter.
- Slowly add the clarified butter into a container, leave all of the milky solids in the bottom of the pot.
- Discard these solids and allow the clarified butter to cool until just warm, this takes about 15 minutes.
- Place a pot with about three inches of water on the medium heat, heating until it simmers.
- Using a stainless steel bowl, add in the yolks along with two teaspoons of cold water and whisk them together until they are foamy and light. This takes about three minutes.

- Add in three or four drops of lemon juice to the yolk mixture and whisk it together for about a minute.

- Set the bowl on top of the pot, making sure that the bottom of the bowl doesn't hit the water.

- Whisk the mixture together until they thicken up, around one to two minutes. Set the bowl off of the simmering water.

- In a very thin stream, add in the clarified butter to the yolk mixture. You need to whisk continuously until you use all of the butter and sauce is thick and smooth. If the butter is added too quickly, the sauce could end up breaking.

- Whisk in the rest of the lemon juice and salt.

- This sauce will have to be used right away, or only let it sit for an hour. Get rid of any that you don't use.

# Conclusion

Thank you for making it through to the end of *Keto Diet for Beginners*. Let's hope it was informative and able to provide you with all of the tools you need to achieve your goals whatever they may be.

You now have all the information you need to begin a successful ketogenic diet. This is a wonderful diet to follow to lose weight and even to maintain your desired weight. While, at first, you may experience some negative side effects, they will go away if you stick with it. It may seem tough, but it's worth it. You will notice results nearly immediately. Now, it's time to get started.

Finally, if you found this book useful in any way, a review on Amazon is always appreciated!

# Description

Something that nearly every person can relate to is struggling to lose weight. This is true if you are looking to lose that stubborn five pounds or if you have a lot of weight to lose. It's frustrating, and there is a nauseating amount of weight loss plans out there. How is a person supposed to be able to figure out how to lose weight when the professionals aren't even sure?

That's where this book and the ketogenic diet come into play. With this book, you will learn everything that you need to know to start a ketogenic diet and lose weight for good. If you scour the internet, you will find a lot of different, conflicting information on the keto diet. Some say it's terrible, some are lukewarm about it, and others believe it is the best weight loss plan ever. Whatever side you take is up to you, but I'm hoping that, with this book, you will learn to love this diet.

In this book, you will learn:

- How to start a ketogenic diet
- A meal plan to help you lose 21 pounds in 21 days
- What ketosis is and why it's so important
- Lots of recipes so that you never go hungry
- The different ketogenic plans
- The side effects that can happen
- What you can eat
- And much more!

The ketogenic diet is more than a weight loss plan. It's a way of life that brings so many more benefits than other weight loss plans. While you may find it difficult when you start the diet, it does get easier. The payoff is worth the effort. Don't wait any longer and get started today.

www.ingramcontent.com/pod-product-compliance
Lightning Source LLC
Chambersburg PA
CBHW081153020426
42333CB00020B/2493